THE
FITNESS
MINDSET

EAT FOR ENERGY, TRAIN FOR TENSION, MANAGE YOUR MINDSET, REAP THE RESULTS

BRIAN KEANE

CONTENTS

INTRODUCTION

When I was about seven years old, I remember watching a talk show with my grandmother and seeing this man with big muscles, who in my eyes looked like a superhero. I recall being engrossed in every word that came out of his mouth and listening to how he used to do hundreds of push-ups in his small bedroom in Austria when he was nine or ten. I remember running to my room to do as many push-ups as I could – which turned out to be maybe one, possibly two! But I went to bed that night dreaming that someday, I would be big, strong and muscular like the man on TV. That man went on to become one of the top grossing movie stars of all time and the Governor of California. His name – Arnold Schwarzenegger. That night, the seed of my love for fitness was sown.

I was born into a massive sporting family and grew up on a small farm in Connemara in the West of Ireland.

I wasn't very scholarly at school: from the age of six to 17 or 18, my entire life circulated around playing sports, especially Gaelic Football, Ireland's national sport, which was my personal favourite.

My closest friends like to joke with me that I'm the living embodiment of, 'If it isn't a priority, it doesn't get done' and there's a lot of truth to this. From an academic stand point I just about got through school, but from a sports standpoint, I made it into every team I tried out for, spending hours every evening practising skills and drills to improve my performance. To master my football techniques, I would learn to kick equally well with both feet, would hang car tyres in front of my home-made goals and try to kick the ball through them. I wouldn't enter the house until I passed the ball through the tyre 10 times in a row. I did everything to improve my game. My schoolbag was a glorified doorstopper for most of my teens.

School was never really a focus for me, so I never excelled until my early twenties. I regularly had teachers tell me I was going to be on welfare for life unless I turned professional in one of the sports I played.

I remember one time when I was picked up by the ear and kicked out of the class for mapping out my workout routine during the time allotted to some other task. I recall walking down the long narrow corridor to the principal's office with my heart in my mouth. It was the third or fourth time I had been sent that week. I'll never forget the conversation we had that day.

My principal, also named Brian, sat me down and told me that although I obviously should be doing the allocated tasks and not calculating my 10 rep max during class, I was going to be fine in life. He had seen my work ethic and dedication to football and talked about my ability to lead others on the pitch. He said that I had the personality to do big things with my life and never to let other teachers' opinions of me change who I am at the core. I don't remember much of the conversation, but I can never forget the feeling I had when I left that office. 'People will forget what you said, people will forget what you did, but people will never forget how you made them feel' (Maya Angelou), and I think even at a subconscious level, that's where my 'just do you' life philosophy comes from. That was the first time I had an authority figure, besides my mum, tell me that I was going to do something with my life, and I'll be forever grateful for the belief that conversation instilled in me. It is rightly said that great teachers can inspire you to do great things.

I've since gone to university, received an honours degree

in Business, completed post-graduation in teaching, won an All-Ireland medal with my club, travelled the world as a professional fitness model and run my own business that works with and serves thousands of people every year.

This book is a culmination of everything I have learnt over the last 17 years of training and nearly 30 years of life. The book is split into two sections.

The first half contains everything about fitness and health: nutrition, training, supplements, sleep, alcohol and hydration. These are the essentials you need to get into incredible shape, increase your energy and reap the results of understanding how your body works. I nearly quit fitness several times during my early twenties from sheer information overload. There was so much conflicting material out there that I didn't know what to believe, what to try or what worked. I've used my personal 17 years of training and nutrition knowledge to try and find a shortcut for your journey. I effectively wrote all this for the 22-year-old me who nearly quit a hundred times.

The second half is focused on cultivating the mindset to get great results, using step-by-step strategies to help you implement them. It discusses everything from creating habits, setting goals and reducing stress to maximise your energy levels, to my own personal stories of dealing with stress, anxiety and worry in my own life.

The last section is entitled 'Practical life tips' and is written for my daughter. None of us truly knows how much time we have on this planet and the life tips are a culmination of personal philosophies that I want to pass on to my daughter in case anything ever happens to me.

HOW TO READ THIS BOOK

Personally, I love being able to flip through books and pick out the most relevant sections for me so I've written this book with that in mind. I have also woven in personal stories to give context to theoretical ideas. If fitness is your primary goal and you are just looking for a blueprint to get into incredible shape, I would definitely recommend starting with Section One. If you are looking for some practical life tips and how to deal with anxiety, stress, worry or any of life's regular problems, I would advise jumping straight to the second section, Mind-set.

However, if you are looking to get in great shape, have more energy, feel better and happier in all aspects of your life and nurture the mind-set to maintain it, then I would read the book in its entirety. Thank you for reading, and I hope this book serves you incredibly well on your journey.

SECTION I
FITNESS

CHAPTER I
NUTRITION

This chapter is designed to give you an improved understanding of how nutrition plays a vital role in giving your body energy, helping it use fat as a fuel source and aiding in building lean muscle. This section discusses everything from calories and macronutrients to the specific role of each in changing your body composition and improving energy levels. We will start with the foundation principles such as 'what is a calorie;' and 'what are macro nutrients' and other ideas that are imperative to understand in order to change your body composition and improve your energy levels.

We will explore the detailed ways in which certain foods affect the body in a positive and negative way (in the context of body composition, fat loss and energy levels) and also investigate the roles of three macro nutrients: protein, carbohydrates and fat in more detail.

NEVER BUILD YOUR HOUSE ON SAND

Personally, I'm not very religious, but I do love the messages from some of the great books of times past, *The Bible*, *The Torah* and the *Quran* to name a few. One of my favourite passages in *The Bible* is from the parable of the wise and the foolish builders in *Matthew* 7:26, which I paraphrase: 'It's a foolish man who builds his house on sand.'

Nutrition is exactly the same. Once you have the fundamentals and a solid foundation for nutrition, it's easy to build on top of that. There are so many different nutritional strategies you can follow: clean eating, keto, IIFYM, Paleo, 80:20, to name just a few, but the key is to get the foundations in place first. I will not offer an opinion regarding which strategy is the best. They all work in their own way and learning which system fits into your lifestyle is always going to be the key. I will, though, recommend the foundation principles that I think every nutritional strategy should have and then you can adopt different systems based on these principles.

Before we dig deeper, it's important that you understand the fundamentals. All great ideas are built on solid foundations, and calories and macronutrients are the foundations of every good nutritional strategy.

WHAT IS A CALORIE?

A calorie (or a kilocalorie) is a unit of energy. Human beings require energy to survive – to breathe, move, pump blood, etc., and we acquire this energy from food.

The number of calories in a food item is a measure of how much potential energy that food possesses.

For example:

1g of carbohydrates has 4 calories
1g of protein has 4 calories
1g of fat has 9 calories

Various foods are a compilation of these three building blocks. Therefore, if you know how many carbohydrates, fats and proteins are present in any given food item, you can calculate how many calories or how much energy that food contains. Below is an example of the formula for calculating the number of calories in a food.

For example:

100g of oats (generic brand)
This is a low-fat, high-carb, low-to-moderate-protein food.
Protein: 16.5g (16.5g × 4 kcal),

Carbohydrates: 66g (66g × 4 kcal),

Fat: 7g (7 g × 9 kcal),

Total calories: 393 kcal.

Note: The same formula can be applied to any food item to calculate the number of calories.

HOW MANY CALORIES DO YOU NEED?

This number can vary greatly from person to person. From the nutritional labels of the foods you buy, you may notice that the 'percent daily values' are based on a 2,000 or 2,500 calorie diet.

According to the National Health Service (NHS), 2,500 (for males) or 2,000 (for females) calories is a rough average of how much a semi-active adult needs to eat in a day. However, your body might need more or less than the recommended number of calories in order to achieve the physique you're striving for. Height, weight, gender, age and activity level, all affect your caloric needs.

In addition, at the most basic level, if you eat more calories than you burn, you will add weight. On the flip side, if you eat fewer calories than you burn, you will lose weight. This is true at the most basic level, but there are a number of other factors that come into play.

1. **The digestion of each food** – One of my mentors would always say to me, 'it's not about what you eat, it's about what you absorb'. The truth is, it's a combination of both. Your food choices are important, but you also need to consider how much of that food you are absorbing. Will 100g of rice from a microwave packet filled with preservatives be absorbed the same way as 100 g of pure rice that needs to be boiled and drained? The answer is 'no.' The removal of some fibre and the addition of preservatives, means that microwavable ready-made foods will have a significantly lower absorption rate than their non-processed alternatives, thus leaving you with less energy for the same number of calories. Further in this chapter, I will discuss how making one simple change – eliminating or greatly reducing processed foods – can have an incredibly beneficial impact on your body's ability to burn body fat or build lean muscle. With this change, you will also experience an extremely noticeable effect in your energy – even after merely a few days.

2. **Keeping the blood sugar levels stable** – As mentioned above, once you hit your daily calorie or macronutrient (macro) targets, in theory, you will lose or gain weight. However, as much as I wish it were as simple as that, your body doesn't work as one plus one

equals two. In my experience, keeping your blood sugars levels stable is one of the most important factors in any nutritional plan. If your blood sugar levels are not balanced, you are going to suffer from low energy levels, mood swings and a general 'high/low' that comes with sugar spikes and crashes. Later in the chapter, I will discuss how balancing blood sugar levels can completely eliminate cravings, improve energy levels and increase your body's ability to burn fat or build lean muscle.

In terms of just losing weight, it can be as simple as eating fewer calories than you burn. If you want to lose weight quickly and you don't care about body composition, muscle tone, energy levels or keeping the weight off over the long term, then by all means you can stop reading right away. However, if you want to know how to eat more real food, increase your energy levels, have a leaner, more toned or muscular physique AND keep it for the long term, then keep reading.

There's one more fundamental that needs to be understood before we continue: macronutrients.

What are macronutrients?

Definition: 'A type of food (e.g. fat, protein, carbohydrate) required in large amounts in the diet.' – *Webster Dictionary.*

Macronutrients are nutrients that provide calories or energy. Nutrients are the substances required for growth, metabolism and for other body functions. Since 'macro' means large, macronutrients are the nutrients required in large amounts.

There are three primary macronutrients:

- Proteins

- Fats

- Carbohydrates

PROTEINS

Proteins are made of varying combinations of amino acids, 20 in all. Amino acids make up every tissue and substance in our bodies, from hair and heart to hormones. Depending on your goals, in order to build a leaner or more muscular body, we need the right combination of amino acids interacting with fundamentally healthy cells in order to repair and build tissues for lean muscle.

Carbohydrates and fats are important, but nothing compares to the ability of amino acids to grow, repair and maintain a healthy tissue.

There are eight essential amino acids for adults (valine, isoleucine, leucine, phenylalanine, threonine, tryptophan, methionine, and lysine) and nine for children (add histidine to the list). The body can make all the other amino acids from the essential ones, but we must get the essential ones from the foods or supplements we consume. This is why it's so important to supplement with leuicine, isoleuicine and valine (Branch Chain Amino Acids) when trying to build lean muscle, as your body can't produce them by itself.

Animal and fish protein contains all the essential amino acids in proper proportions to one another – a characteristic of all flesh foods – and thus is known as complete protein. You can also get essential amino acids in the plant kingdom. They are just not in their complete protein proportions, and therefore, you have to mix and match them to make them complete proteins. Because most plants provide inadequate amounts of certain amino acids in relation to others, plant protein is normally referred to as 'incomplete' protein.

Why do we need protein?

- Growth: especially when looking to build lean muscle tissue.

- Tissue repair: to repair muscle tissue after intensive workouts.

- Immune function: to avoid getting sick.

- To get energy when carbohydrate is not available: This is by gluconeogenesis, whereby your body converts protein to glucose for energy.

- To preserve lean muscle mass: to retain the muscle you already have.

How do I get my protein if I don't eat meat?

It's true that meat and eggs are complete proteins, in contrast to beans and nuts. However, we don't need every essential amino acid from every meal we eat – we only need a sufficient amount of each amino acid each day. During the digestive process, our bodies free the amino acids present in our food and create other substances from them. According to the Centres for Disease Control and Prevention, if something we eat doesn't contain all the essential amino acids required by the body, we have a small window (about a day) to ingest the complementary ones to complete the amino-acid equation.

The body doesn't house or store amino acids (i.e. you need to eat them every day), but as long as you eat the correct food combinations during the day, you will be fine. As mentioned above, you don't necessarily have to combine them in one meal. You just need to make sure that you combine the right foods to get all the essential amino acids in the right amounts by the end of the day. There are numerous ways to use food combinations to get all your essential amino acids. I'll list a few examples below.

Combining nuts and seeds with legumes or grains

Combining legumes with sunflower seeds, sesame seeds or nuts such as walnuts, almonds or cashew provides complete proteins. One of my personal favourites is a trail mix of nuts, cashews, sunflower seeds with hummus or guacamole dip and raw vegetables.

To cement the idea that you do not need to consume protein-rich food together in a single meal to reap the benefits of combining proteins, The University of Michigan's reports show that, 'Eating a variety of foods with incomplete proteins throughout the day allows your body to get the amino acids you need from diet.' The one thing to remember is that your body doesn't store complete proteins for a rainy day. According to the Standing Committee on the Scientific Evaluation for Dietary Reference Intakes, 'There is no evidence for a protein reserve that serves only as a store to meet future needs', which means you need to stay on top of your nutrition and combine your foods every single day to reap all the benefit of essential amino acids. However, once you use the correct nutritional strategy that includes all the essential amino acids, you can get all the benefits of a complete protein eater, so long as you are resourceful with your combinations.

The benefits of animal products

The truth is, it's significantly easier to get all your essential amino acids from meat, fish and eggs, which are already loaded with them all. While steak contains protein, it also contains fat, vitamins A, B, iron and zinc. However, not all meat and fish are created equally. Different animal proteins have different nutritional densities. The differences between a grass-fed cow or a free-range chicken and an antibiotic-pumped cow and factory chicken are tremendous.

Avoid factory-farmed meat and fish

The most nutrient-rich proteins are from properly raised meat. Personally, I'm a massive fan of poultry, but the hormone-loaded chickens that are found in some commercial supermarkets are best avoided. If you can get your hands on organic and/or free-range chicken (just ask your local butcher), you are going to get a much higher nutritional return.

In case of fish, try to avoid farmed fish that has been pumped full of colourings, and opt for wild fish whenever possible. Again, your supermarket or local fishmonger should be able to tell you which fish is wild and which has been farmed. There's a frustrating paradox for those who eat farmed fish for their health, as the nutritional benefits of farmed fish are greatly decreased.

Take omega 3 fatty acids. Wild fish get their omega 3 from aquatic plants. Farmed fish, however, are often fed corn, soy or other feed stuff that have little or no omega 3s. The unnatural, high-corn diet also means that some farmed fish accumulate unhealthy levels of the wrong fatty acids. The most concerning issue is that farmed fish are routinely dosed with antibiotics, which can then enter your body and cause all kinds of harm, not to mention slowing down any physical progress, such as losing fat, building muscle, etc. Remember the famous quote, 'You are what you eat'? You can probably extend this to, 'You are also what your food eats.'

Eat the right meat and get more vitamin B12

Vitamin B12 is a water-soluble vitamin that keeps your nerves and blood cells healthy. It is responsible for the smooth functioning of several critical body processes. It is pretty easy to develop a vitamin B12 deficiency, the first symptom normally being chronic fatigue.

Strict vegetarians or vegans, heavy drinkers and smokers are usually most susceptible to vitamin B12 deficiency.

B12 is found only in animal products, yet even lacto-ovo vegetarians (those who drink milk and eat eggs) may miss out on it. Sometimes what matters the most isn't whether a nutrient is found within a food, but whether the body can actually absorb it and use it properly. According to the report in the *Journal of Experimental Biology and Medicine*, the bioavailability (how much you absorb) of vitamin B12 from eggs is less than 9%, which means that from all the B12 found in eggs, the body absorbs only 9%. Compare this to red meat for example, which has a bioavailability as high as 77%. That's not to say that eggs are not incredibly nutritious because they are, the yolks in particular, but B12 isn't their strong suit.

If you are a vegetarian, vegan, smoker or drinker, you should seriously consider adding B12 to your supplement regimen. Personally, I use vitamin B12 spray every single day for the regulation of my nervous system, which can also reduce stress, worry and anxiety. However, there are numerous other benefits to adding B12 to your supplement regimen if you are not consuming it from food.

- It is required to convert carbohydrates into glucose in the body, thus leading to energy production and a decrease in fatigue and lethargy in the body. Basically, it massively reduces your risk of chronic fatigue.

- It helps maintain a healthy digestive system. Remember, it's more about what you absorb than what you eat.

- It is essential for healthy skin, hair and nails and can help in cell reproduction and constant renewal of the skin.

- It has been thought to help prevent breast, colon, lung and prostate cancer through regulation of the nervous system.

Our body can store and recycle B12, an evolutionary adaption that makes sense, as B12 is so necessary that our bodies have evolved the capacity to store it for survival in times of scarcity. However, there's a downside to being able to store and recycle it: the symptoms of long-term inadequate intake can take years to show themselves. Long-term deficiency puts you at a risk of nerve degeneration, mental disturbance and depression amongst a host of other problems.

Once these symptoms manifest, it's nearly impossible

to fully recover. The take-home message is to make sure that you get enough vitamin B12 from your meat or consider adding it to your supplement regimen. Personally, I only eat red meat once or twice a week, so I hedge my bets and supplement with it.

'An ounce of prevention is
worth a pound of cure'

BEN FRANKLIN

How to choose your eggs

The old adage, 'You are what you eat' certainly holds true when considering the nutritional value of eggs. For chicken to be classified as 'free range', it must have been granted access to the outdoors during the raising process. Hens that have access to better pasture have better eggs than birds kept in cages.

Free-range hens eat a healthy, natural diet that then manifests into healthier and more nutritious eggs. Alongside having more vitamin A and vitamin E, the main benefit of free-range eggs is their omega 3 fatty acid value.

As mentioned in the fat section of the book, omega 3s are an essential fatty acid because the body can't manufacture it on its own, and you must consume it from food. According to Barb Gorski from Sustainable Agriculture Research and Education, free-range hens normally produce four times the omega 3s as their caged sisters. The egg yolk, which has most of the nutritional value, is the best indicator of egg quality. A darker yolk, normally dark orange, is an indication of a chicken fed with nutritious and balanced diet rich in omega 3, while a bright yellow yolk is normally the result of caged, poorly fed chickens.

Free-range organic chicken farmers must feed their chickens lots of fresh greens including kale, collard and broccoli to produce the dark orange yolk, which has been proven to not only taste richer but also being richer in nutrients and vitamins.

The take-home message is to always buy free-range organic eggs, which are slightly more expensive, but pack a much higher nutritional punch and can actually help you get leaner, faster, due to their higher omega 3 levels.

What are the best sources of protein?

Personally, I prefer meat and fish sources, as they already have all the essential amino acids that your body requires, but even if you don't eat meat, you can get all your essential amino acids by combining the right foods. It just means you have to get a bit more experimental with your recipes.

I'll list my favourites below. Personally, I try and source all my meat and fish from local butchers and fishmongers, as they can tell me if they have used any antibiotics, hormones or additives. However, most supermarkets also have organic, free-range or grass-fed sections. Again, they may cost a little bit more (but not in all cases – my local butcher is actually cheaper than most supermarkets) so shop around and find what works the best for you.

Some foods such as beef and salmon also have a high-fat content, but are primarily protein foods, which is why I have included them in this list.

- Chicken (free range if possible)
- Turkey (free range if possible)
- Free-range eggs
- Beef or lamb (grass fed if possible)
- Rice protein powder
- Whey protein powder
- Wild fish (salmon, cod, mackerel, etc.)

FAT

Thankfully, over the past two decades, we have begun to move away from the 'Fat is bad for you' or 'Fat will make you fat' mindset, which has negatively affected so many people's lives, energy levels and waistlines. With the massive influx of processed foods and refined cereals over the past decade, unless you are actually going out of your way to consume good healthy fat, you're very likely to be undereating it.

Why do we need fat?

- For brain function: Omega 3, for example, plays a critical role in brain function.

- To burn body fat: Certain types of fats such as conjugated linoleic acid (CLA) found in grass-fed cows and pasteurised butter can actually help your body burn fat.

- For steady energy: Fat is the most concentrated source of energy. It can give you steady energy throughout the day and keep your blood sugar levels stable.

- To absorb certain vitamins: Vitamins A, D, E, K and carotenoids are all fat soluble, i.e. you need to consume them with fat for their absorption.

- Protection: Actual body fat can provide cushioning for the organs.

Eating the right kind of fat is absolutely vital for optimal health.

Dietary fats for repair and growth

Fatty acids have a profound effect on muscle gain, fat loss and overall health. Fat is the building block of all cell membranes. It is also the precursor for all natural steroid hormones and some neurotransmitters (a 'precursor' is a substance from which another substance is formed, similar to putting all the ingredients for a cake into the oven in order to make the actual cake.)

Most importantly, certain fatty acids can generate a hormone-like effect on the body, regulating hunger, fat loss and muscle-building hormones. This is the primary reason why some modern-day diets can completely ruin your metabolism. Modern breakfast cereals and cereal bars for example are so highly processed, high in sugar and devoid of absorbable nutrients that they leave you fighting a losing blood sugar battle for the rest of the day. The answer is to eat more fat.

Define fat

When we talk about fat types – saturated, monounsaturated and polyunsaturated – we're actually talking about fatty acids. Fatty acids are chains of carbon and hydrogen atoms attached to a carboxyl group (think of it like a hinge on your bike that keeps individual chain links together.) Every fat, whether plant or animal, is made up of these same raw materials.

In saturated fat, every link in the fatty acid chain is secured – it's saturated. Monounsaturated fats have just one unsecured link (mono is Latin for 'one'), and polyunsaturated fats have two or more unsecured links in their chains (poly is Latin for 'many').

In truth, almost all the natural fats we eat are a blend of these three kinds of fat, but whatever a fat is mostly made of, whether saturated, monounsaturated or polyunsaturated fat, is generally what we call it. We do the same with macronutrients. Oats, for example, have a little fat and some protein, but are primarily comprised of carbohydrates, which is why we label them as a 'carbohydrate' food.

Avoid margarines and eat egg yolks and real butter

Saturated fat was demonized during the early 90's because we thought it raised cholesterol, and we linked high cholesterol to heart disease.

The heart disease epidemic is a relatively new problem in human history, and according to the author of *Eat the Yolks*, Liz Wolfe, 'The first recorded heart attack was in 1912 and by 1930 the number of heart attacks had reached 3,000 and by 1960, there were over 500,000 deaths recorded from heart attacks.'

People were terrified and needed an explanation, and a bad guy. In stepped saturated fat. The western culture's panic led to the development of two ideas that became interlinked: saturated fat is bad, and saturated fat raises cholesterol levels, which gives you a heart attack. This is where margarines and vegetable oil came in to save the day.

According to Chris Masterjob, an expert in nutrition science, randomised controlled trials have shown that polyunsaturated fats can't reduce heart diseases. In fact, no study on replacing animal fat (saturated fat) with plant-based polyunsaturated fat has shown to reduce mortality. More interestingly, Masterjob stated that these studies showed 'An increased risk of cancer after five years and possible increase in heart disease risk'.

Are these heart-healthy vegetable oils therefore bad for us? I'll let you make your own decision regarding this, but if fat loss, muscle building or increasing energy is your goal, margarines and other vegetable oils are very unlikely to support you on your journey. It's also worth noting that the vegetable oils are made up of corn, soya and canola. Corn is a grain, not a vegetable. Soybeans are legumes, not vegetables. Canola is derived from a seed, not a vegetable.

As mentioned earlier, in the case of eggs, the nutritional density of the egg yolk of a free-range chicken to that of her sister raised in a cage or a factory is also worlds apart.

Considering that margarine is generally a blend of crops oils and usually includes additives like emulsifiers, and that butter from pastured cows actually contains fat-burning ingredients like CLA (which is present in most fat-burning supplements), it's probably better to stick to the real thing. Kerrygold Irish butter for example is produced from pastured cows.

The key with fat is to make sure you don't eat too much, as it is calorie dense (i.e. you don't need to eat a lot to get a lot of calories), but factoring it into your nutritional plan can make you feel more satiated, give you more energy and can actually speed up fat loss in conjunction with the right training program and overall nutritional plan.

But what about calories?

Having an idea of calorie consumption is important for your fitness goals. If you want to lose weight and your calorie maintenance, which is the number of calories you need to eat to stay the same weight, is 2,000 kcal, and you eat 6,000 kcal every day, you will probably not lose weight or body fat too quickly. On the other hand, if you are trying to build muscle and your maintenance is 2,000 kcal, you need to eat significantly more in order to build lean muscle. However, the amount is obviously dependent on the speed of your metabolism, current body fat levels, general lifestyle, amongst other factors.

Fat has more calories per gram (9 kcal) than either carbs or protein (both 4 kcal). However, the reality is that 500 kcal from fat is absorbed much differently than 500 kcal from carbohydrates. Fat is more satiating, meaning it will leave you feeling fuller for longer, and including good quality fats that help stabilize blood sugar and hunger levels can be the key to losing body fat, building more muscle and giving you steady energy throughout the day.

Eat fat, lose fat

The take-home message is pretty simple. Eat real food.

Our bodies and digestive systems are designed to eat food as near to its natural state as possible, and not the low-fat versions. Therefore, eat properly raised animals, minimally processed animal products and wild fish, and as long as you have calculated the amount of calories you are eating, don't fear the fat that comes with them.

Not all fat is created equal

One of the biggest misconceptions that I fell victim to in my early twenties was that, 'Eating fat will make you fat'. I think a more accurate rephrasing would be, 'Certain fat will make you fat'. The three main types of fat that are important to understand are omega 6, omega 3 and trans fatty acids.

Omega 3 and omega 6

Both essential fatty acids (EFA), omega 3 and omega 6 are considered vital and beneficial. However, omega 3 EFA is normally considered slightly more important, as the modern western diet is likely to be more deficient in omega 3 than omega 6. This is because the king of the omega 3 family, alpha-linolenic acid (ALA), and his metabolically active prince and princess, eicosapentaenoic acid (EPA) and docosahexaenoic acid (DHA), are more unsaturated and prone to damage in cooking and food processing.

In other sections of the book, I've spoken how food processing removes a lot of nutrients from food, and omega 3 is a primary example.

Why do I need omega 3?

Omega 3 is actively involved in critical biological functions such as improving cognitive abilities, helping you retain information better, helping you perform complicated tasks more effectively, alleviating pain and inflammation, and improving insulin sensitivity.

If you find that you have brain fog, pain from inflammation or have body fat to lose, it might be worth increasing your omega 3 intake.

The best sources of omega 3

The best seed oils for omega 3 are flax (also known as linseed), hemp and pumpkin. For example, one of my favourite health shakes includes a mixture of rice or whey protein, flaxseed oil, hempseeds and pumpkin seeds.

If you eat carnivorous fish such as mackerel, herring, tuna and salmon, or their oils, you can bypass the conversion stage of alpha linoleic acid and go straight to EPA and DHA. This is why fish-eating cultures (the Japanese culture for example) have three times the omega 3 than their western counterparts. Vegans who eat more seeds tend to have much higher levels of omega 3 as well.

What are the best sources of fat?

- Oily fish (salmon, mackerel)

- Nuts (almonds, walnuts, cashews)

- Seeds (pumpkin, linseed, chia)

- Oils (flaxseed, hemp)

Avoid this type of fat or you *will* get fat

Trans-fatty acids or 'trans fats' definition:

> 'An unsaturated fatty acid of a type occurring in margarines and manufactured cooking oils as a result of the hydrogenations process. Consumption of such acids is thought to increase the risk of atherosclerosis (a disease of the arteries).'
>
> **WEBSTER DICTIONARY**

Trans fats are created as a result of the partial hydrogenation process, or as Liz Wolfe describes it, 'The process of beating an already unhealthy oil into partially hydrogenated submission'. This basically means they change already unhealthy oils into something even worse! Not only have trans fats been shown to lead to a range of health problems (heart disease, obesity etc.), but they are also the single worst types of fats if you are trying to reduce your own levels of body fat. Your body can store them pretty easily.

To understand how bad trans fats truly are, here's a brief explanation at its simplest form of how your body actually taps into fat stores, burning through unwanted body fat in the process.

There are obviously digestive, metabolic and hormonal processes that affect this, but at the most basic level your body's preferred source of energy is glucose (all carbohydrates you consume get converted to glucose). To simplify, any excess glucose gets stored as glycogen (stored carbohydrate), and then any excess glucose gets stored as body fat (fat stores). Following is the energy chain.

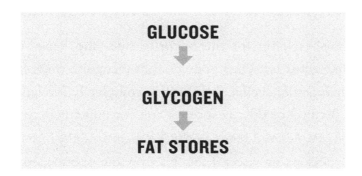

GLUCOSE

⬇

GLYCOGEN

⬇

FAT STORES

Now, add trans fats into the mix and observe how the energy chain changes.

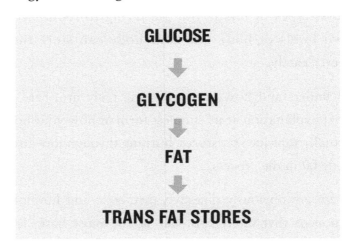

GLUCOSE

⬇

GLYCOGEN

⬇

FAT

⬇

TRANS FAT STORES

You have now added another figurative 'wall' to jump over in your quest to lose body fat. Personally, when I used to eat fast food, hydrogenated oils and other trans fatty acids, it normally increased body fat around my 'stubborn areas' (i.e. places you struggle to remove fat from) such as my lower abdomen and glute region.

'Trans' is Latin for the opposite side, and hence the name trans fat. Your body doesn't recognise trans fats – their actual chemical makeup is completely foreign to it. Because of this, as soon as you consume them, your body panics and tends to shuttle them straight into the fat pockets or visceral fat (fat over the organs), so as not to damage your vital organs.

This is basically a survival safety mechanism: your vital organs are safe if the 'unknown' consumption – trans fats in this case – are safely tucked away in your fat pockets. The easiest way to avoid trans fats is to reduce or eliminate deep fat fried or fast food alongside certain margarines. Not only will you get a substantial increase in energy levels, but your process of reducing unwanted body fat will also significantly speed up.

CARBOHYDRATES

The human body is designed to run on carbohydrates. While we can use protein and fat for energy, the easiest fuels for our body to use are carbohydrates.

When we eat complex carbohydrates like wholegrains, vegetables, beans and lentils, or simpler carbohydrates like fruit, the body does exactly what it is designed to do: it breaks them down and gives us energy. Even better, as these foods haven't been modified or processed, all the nutrients that the body needs for digestion and metabolism are already present in them. They also contain fibre, which is a less digestible type of carbohydrate that helps the digestive system run smoothly.

Carbohydrates have developed a pretty bad reputation over recent years, but when used correctly, they can be massively beneficial in keeping blood sugar stable and energy levels constant and fuelling your body for workouts.

Remember, carbohydrates have one job – to give you energy. There is no 'essential carbohydrate' like essential amino acids from protein or essential fatty acids from fat: they exist to give your body and brain energy. Keeping this in mind, their correct use can be a great weapon in your arsenal. I like to think of carbohydrates like a guard dog – if you treat them well throughout their life, they will look after you, make you feel better and help you sleep better at night. If you abuse them though, they can turn around and bite you just as fast.

Why do we need carbohydrates?

As mentioned above, we don't 'need' carbohydrates. However, if you are a highly active individual, carbohydrates will definitely have some great benefits for your body.

- Body's main source of fuel: glucose and glycogen.

- Easily used by the body for energy: fuelling intensive workouts.

- Used by all tissues and cells for energy: glucose.

- Can be stored in the muscles and liver and later used for energy.

  Note: This is great for fitness-seeking people for whom performance is key, but overdoing it can also lead to fat gain.

- Good source of fibre: certain types of carbohydrates that our body can't digest are passed through the intestinal tract intact and help to move waste out of the body.

Are fruits good or bad?

Unlike vegetables, particularly green leafy vegetables, which are nearly impossible to overeat, the answers regarding the effect of fruit on body composition can vary depending on who you speak with. I have heard every argument from 'Fruit will make you fat' to 'We're evolved to eat fruit, which should be a staple part of every diet on the planet!'. There are a few topics, which I can argue just as strongly on both sides.

On one hand, I am a massive fan of the vitamins and minerals that fruits naturally contain. In addition, if timed right, they can balance blood sugar and enormously curb a natural sweet tooth. On the other hand, fructose is converted to glucose pretty easily and excess of it can lead to unnecessary fat gain. Further, there are certain fruits that are nearly pure glucose and can hugely elevate blood sugar levels, leading to a whole host of energy crashes and fat-gain problems. The truth isn't whether fruits are inherently good or bad; it's the selection choices you make and their timings that are key.

Fruits contain a simple sugar called fructose, which needs no digestion and can therefore enter the bloodstream quickly, like glucose or sucrose. However, unlike them, fructose is classified as slow releasing because the body can't use it as it is and has to convert it into glucose before your body can effectively use it. This slows down the sugar's effect on the metabolism.

Some fruits such as grapes, mangoes and dates contain pure glucose and are therefore faster releasing. Bananas contain both fructose and glucose and thereby raise blood sugar levels quite speedily and are thus worth watching out for too.

Through personal experience, the negatives of raising blood sugar dramatically, even post workout, massively outweighs the benefits. It feels as if you are spending the rest of the day trying to stabilise your energy levels as your blood sugars balance. I would use these fruits in moderation to avoid an imbalance in blood sugars, which can slow down the fat-burning process and lead to unnecessary energy drops during the day.

Avoid refined carbohydrates

Refined carbohydrates such as white bread, white rice or refined cereals have a similar effect to refined sugar. When you eat simple carbohydrates, you get a rapid increase in blood sugar level and a corresponding surge in energy. A drop however follows the surge, as the body scrambles to balance your blood sugar levels. This drop, especially if it happens frequently through the day, can give you a whole host of problems, right from short-term problems like irritability, tiredness and headaches to long-term problems like fatigue and weight gain. This is where balancing your blood sugar levels becomes the key.

Balancing blood sugars

Keeping blood sugar balanced is probably the most important factor in maintaining steady energy levels and weight. The level of glucose in your blood largely determines your appetite. When the level of glucose drops, you feel hungry. The glucose in your bloodstream is available for your cells to produce energy. When the levels are too high, the body converts the excess to glycogen or fat, our long-term energy reserves. If our blood sugar levels are too low, we experience a host of symptoms including fatigue, poor concentration, irritability, depression, headaches and digestive problems. So how do we keep our blood sugars balanced?

Four tips to keep blood sugar levels balanced

1. **Eat something small every three hours:** A great breakdown is to have your three main meals, breakfast, lunch and dinner, with two or three snacks in between. Keeping your energy and blood sugar levels stable and in balance can allow you to train harder without getting food cravings associated with blood sugar drops, which can come from missing meals and snacks. This can give you a significantly better quality of life by increasing your overall energy levels, as a result helping you lose body fat and/or building lean muscle in the process.

2. **Avoid processed food and eat more vegetables:** Processed food actually has two major negative effects on your body. Firstly, ingredients and nutrients from the original source are removed to produce most processed foods and replaced with sugar for preservation. Blood sugars dramatically rise with consumption of these types of food.

   Secondly, the 'energy surge/drop feedback loop' (loads of energy followed by a crash) that refined sugar creates, can have a highly negative effect on your blood sugar levels. If blood sugar levels are out of balance, your entire body will be less efficient at converting carbohydrate for energy. Some can get a mild to severe form of insulin resistance leading to a lack of nutrient uptake for healthy nerve and muscle cells, which can have a detrimental impact on any fat loss and/or muscle building goals.

Vegetables, on top of being very low in calories, are also packed with vitamins, minerals and fibre. I would recommend adding some vegetables or salad to your main meals or eat them as snacks throughout the day.

3. **Eat more fat:** As discussed at length in the fat section above, having a higher level of fat particularly healthy fat like omega 3 from oily fish can do a tremendous job at balancing blood sugar levels. The truth is, if you only eat a diet with good, hormone-boosting fats, nutrient-dense vegetables and quality-protein sources, because fat is satiating and slow releasing, it is unlikely that you would ever have a blood sugar issue. For the majority of people, including myself, this isn't feasible and the key, therefore, is to choose the correct sources of carbohydrate, timing them right and making them work for you.

4. **Eat slow-releasing carbohydrates at insulin-sensitive times:** There are two times in the day (morning and post workout) when you will be particularly insulin sensitive because your body will be more likely to use carbohydrates efficiently and not store them as fat. This varies according to your metabolism but in general, your body will absorb and uptake carbohydrates more efficiently first thing in the morning, after a fasted sleep and post workout, after you have trained.

If you have ever thought to yourself, 'Carbs will make me fat' I will try to crush that myth now. It is true that excess carbohydrates, especially refined sugars and processed carbohydrates, can get transported by the liver and get converted to body fat. However, if you follow a good training program, using short bursts of high-intensity interval training (HIIT) for your cardio and are consuming calories in alignment with your goals, the consumption of good-quality carbohydrates is highly unlikely to increase your body fat.

What are the best sources of carbohydrates?

- Oats

- Sweet potato

- Baby new potatoes

- Brown or basmati rice

- Vegetables

- Fruit (used in alignment with your goals)

As mentioned above, the key is timing your meals to keep your blood sugar levels stable and then using quality food to keep your body fuelled. Here is a sample daily layout, but you can use your own favourite foods to make it suit your lifestyle.

SAMPLE DAILY MENU

BREAKFAST

7:00am: 50g porridge oats and two free-range poached eggs

MORNING SNACK

10:00am: 100g Greek yoghurt and 1 teaspoon of pumpkin seeds

LUNCH

1:00pm: 200g wild salmon, unlimited broccoli and spinach

MID-AFTERNOON SNACK

4:00pm: handful of almonds

DINNER

7:00pm: 150g sweet potato, 150g free-range chicken and 200g roasted carrots

BEFORE-BED SNACK

10:00pm: 1 scoop of whey protein.

CHAPER 2
SUPPLEMENTS

Supplement definition:

> 'A thing added to something else in order
> to complete or enhance it.'
>
> **WEBSTER DICTIONARY**

Supplements make it much easier to get the necessary nutrients to build muscle and lose body fat, and they can give you an advantage and enhance your training when taken the right way, combined with a good diet.

However, using supplements without a good diet is like using amazing motor oil for your car, but forgetting to put the fuel in.

Choosing supplements can be an absolute minefield, with so many products, brands and choices being available today that it's easy to go wrong when making a selection. I've narrowed it down to the absolute essentials that I have used with thousands of clients over the years and which are the most scientifically backed in the market.

The key point to remember when buying supplements is to look at the ingredients and not the brand. There are hundreds of great brands and some not-so-great brands out there, but as long as the product you're looking for has the ingredients below in the correct dosage, they should work well for you.

Furthermore, you should always choose your supplements based on your goals and not your gender. If you are a man or a woman looking to lose body fat, the same supplements will support you, but the dosage may be different.

MUSCLE-BUILDING SUPPLEMENTS

1. Whey protein

The numerous benefits of whey protein include increase in muscular strength and size, decrease in body fat and a faster recovery time.

Muscle protein synthesis is a scientific phrase thrown around a lot, which basically means that this synthesis enables muscle growth and is an important process for increasing muscle size and strength.

Resistance training alone can increase rates of protein synthesis. However, it also increases rates of protein breakdown. For muscle growth to occur, you need to tip the scale in favour of protein synthesis while trying to minimize the breakdown.

Consuming whey protein post workout can substantially increase muscle protein synthesis. Whey protein is a fast-digesting protein that enters the bloodstream rapidly. This allows it to get to your muscles faster and create a bigger spike in protein synthesis compared to food sources.

Dosage: The amount you use can vary depending on your body weight and protein requirements, but 25–50g per serving for men and 10–25g per serving for women 30 minutes after exercise is a good starting point.

2. Creatine

Creatine is the most scientifically researched supplement on the planet. Without going too much into the science, creatine plays a vital role in cellular energy production, as creatine phosphate (phosphocreatine), by regenerating adenosine triphosphate (ATP) in skeletal muscles. ATP is what allows your muscle to contract when you work out.

One of the main functions of creatine is to pull water underneath the muscle. This works similar to filling a plastic water bottle – if you press down hard, the bottle will bend and crack, whereas if you fill it with water, it becomes much harder to bend and crack it. The presence of creatine in muscles has a similar effect.

If you have more water underneath the muscle, as creatine allows, your muscle becomes more durable, meaning you can push or pull more weight or do the same weight for more reps, leading to more fibre tears, which in turn can lead to more lean muscle growth.

There are many forms of creatine, monohydrate, ethyl-ester and tri-malate just to name a few, but they're all essentially creatine, with or without a different ester attached.

Dosage: *Depending on the form, a good starting point is 3–5g pre- and post-workout for men and 1.5–3g for women.*

3. Branch Chain Amino Acids (BCAAs)

The BCAAs are made up of three essential amino acids: leucine, isoleucine and valine. They are essential because the body is unable to produce them from other amino acids, so they must be ingested through food or supplements.

A large percentage of dietary amino acids are oxidized and wasted even before reaching the circulatory system. The exceptions to this pattern are the BCAAs: over 80% of dietary content of leucine, valine and isoleucine reaches circulation.

Whey protein is naturally high in BCAAs, but adding another 3–10g depending on your bodyweight before, during or after your workouts can tremendously improve your recovery.

- -

Dosage: *The dose varies depending on your bodyweight and training program, but a good starting point is 5–10g pre- or post-workout for men and 3–5g for women.*

FAT-BURNING SUPPLEMENTS

Fat burners can effectively aid fat loss when used properly. You must have heard of fat burner pills that can make fat melt off your body. Unfortunately, they don't actually work that way. Fat burners are supplements. They're designed with ingredients that can give you an extra boost to help burn fat. However, they can't replace a good nutritional strategy.

Think of fat burners like a scope on a sniper rifle, only in this case you're trying to shrink fat cells. Diet is the gun, the heavy artillery, and exercise is the firepower. Fat burners may help you aim a bit better and kill fat more efficiently. However, fat burners don't work to their best effect when they're used improperly. They're the figurative 'icing on the cake'. So, which fat burners should you use?

1. Caffeine

Caffeine is a staple ingredient in many popular fat-burning and pre-workout supplements. It primarily helps you lose body fat in two ways:

1. **By boosting your metabolism**: Ingesting caffeine jump-starts the process of lipolysis, which is when your body releases free fatty acids into the bloodstream to be used for energy. In other words, caffeine boosts your metabolism and can help you burn fat.

2. **By giving you an energy boost**: If there's one thing that everyone knows about coffee and caffeinated drinks or pills is that caffeine

is a pretty strong stimulant. It increases alertness and wards off drowsiness temporarily, which means you can perform certain tasks more efficiently for longer on caffeine.

This applies for physical tasks as well as mental tasks. This means a little shot of caffeine can give you the energy you need to give 100% during your workout. And giving 100% in the gym means you'll get the results you want more quickly.

Dosage: *If you don't regularly ingest a lot of caffeine, a couple of hundred milligrams or a strong cup of black coffee will likely produce noticeable effects. You may want to start with 100mg to see how it goes and then up your intake to 200mg. You can then increase the dose by 50mg if you're still not experiencing any effects. Do be careful not to overdo it as the side effects of a caffeine overdose can range from anxiety and insomnia to death.*

Take 30 minutes before your workout to release free fatty acids to be burnt while you train and to increase physical and mental alertness. However, be aware that caffeine has just over a five-hour half-life so if you take it too late at night, it can negatively affect your sleep. This means that if you consume 200mg of caffeine at 12 midday, 100mg will still be in your system at 5pm.

2. Green tea extract

Green tea extract is probably my favourite fat-burning supplement. It has a low-to-moderate dose of caffeine, and it has another ace up its sleeve – polyphenols. These incredible polyphenols are vital for any person trying to get lean.

In the scientific community, polyphenols are more commonly known as flavanols or catechins.

The main catechins in green tea are epicatechin, epicatechin—3-gallate, epigallocatechin, and the one with the highest concentration, epigallocatechin-3-gallate or **EGCG.**

EGCG at a level of 45% or more (the percentage is on the ingredient list of every green tea extract supplement) has the ability to:

- increase 24-hour energy expenditure, burning more calories throughout the day;

- increase the body's key fat-burning hormone, norepinephrine, increasing the rate of fatty acid mobilization;

- prolong thermogenesis, increasing core temperature to burn more calories;

- provide powerful antioxidants; and

- support a healthy immune system, stopping you from getting sick.

Dosage: *For both men and women, taking between 500 mg and 1000 mg of green tea extract (with 45% or more ECGC) first thing in the morning or 30 minutes before training will support fatty acid mobilization and increase metabolism for the rest of the day.*

3. L-Carnitine tartrate

L-carnitine plays an essential role in transporting fat into mitochondria – the furnace of the cell, where it can be burnt for fuel, which basically means it moves fat from the back of the queue to the front to be used as an energy source.

Without adequate L-carnitine, most dietary fats can't get into the mitochondria and be burned for fuel. This is one reason why L-carnitine is considered a 'conditionally essential' nutrient – your body produces it, but if it doesn't produce enough, your fat loss can get seriously affected.

Supplementing with L-carnitine alongside caffeine and green tea extract can dramatically speed up your fat-loss goals without having too much of a 'negative' effect on your central nervous system. If you think of your metabolism as a fire, caffeine and green tea extract make the fire burn brighter, and l-carnitine pushes the fat into the fire to be burnt as fuel.

Dosage: *For both men and women, taking between 1000mg and 3000mg of l-carnitine tartrate first thing in the morning or 30 minutes before training can work very effectively.*

CHAPTER 3
SLEEP

Sleep better and boost your energy

As someone who has been a notoriously poor sleeper most of my life, I find it very easy to see how easily poor sleep quality can affect people's everyday lives. Poor sleep can affect everything from your energy levels to your willpower, and from talking with large groups of people over the years, I've noticed that a large amount of people have very poor sleep fitness.

We waste time falling asleep and spend hours in a light sleep state, which doesn't have the same body and brain boosting benefits of deep and REM sleep. In the past, I would spend an hour trying to fall asleep because my brain wouldn't stop rehashing the day's events or would dwell on what was coming up the next day.

I tried different supplements, going to bed earlier, going to bed later, but I would wake up every morning still groggy. Sleep began to feel like a waste of time. Not only would I lose an hour every night tossing and turning, I wouldn't feel any fresher in the morning and would feel like a zombie until I had my first cup of coffee.

I'm not a sleep doctor, but I have spent years trying to figure out why I wasn't able to sleep better, and this allowed me to learn more about actual sleep quality over sleep quantity. This is determined by how much time you spend in actual REM and delta (deep, restorative) sleep.

Nutrition and sleep

Sleep is important because there is actually a direct link between your diet and sleep. What you eat, directly affects how well you sleep. The quality of your sleep also has a dramatic impact on your energy levels. Naturopathic physician and founder of Biohealth Diagnostics in San Diego, California Reed Davis talks about how 'unless people get to bed by 10:30pm and get a full eight hours of sleep, they're wasting their money'. His philosophy is based on the 'circadian cycle', which is a natural physiological cycle of about 24 hours that persists even in the absence of external cues, i.e. the way we're designed to sleep based on daylight and nightfall – our body clock so to speak.

I noticed that on nights when I got five hours sleep or less, I felt groggy and tired and needed caffeine to get me going. Pretty standard, right? But the same thing happened on the nights I got 10 hours sleep or more.

In contrast, something very interesting happened when I 'split the difference' and got seven-and-a-half or eight hours of sleep. I felt great! If I went to bed at 11pm and set an alarm for 6:30am, I found that I normally woke up before my alarm and felt ready for the day. I tested this for three or four months and found that I had more energy through the day and didn't need a nap (as I had done frequently in previous years) and I could function optimally until about 9:30pm. At this time, I would normally start to unwind for bed.

Why seven-and-a-half hours?

We've all been told, 'You need to get at least eight hours of sleep every night', but why? Admittedly, I try and go to bed for 10:30pm to give myself about half-an-hour to unwind. I normally read something that switches my mind off, and then have lights out for 11:00pm. But I had to ask myself why I feel so much better and have much more energy with seven-and-a-half hours of sleep over, say 10 hours.

After a couple of hours, we enter the dream state sleep, known as rapid eye movement (REM) stage 1. REM sleep normally occurs 90 minutes after the onset of sleep, according to Dr Patrick Holford, author of *Optimum Nutrition for the Mind*. If we are sleep deprived, it may occur within 30 minutes.

We have about four or more REM periods per night, and they go in 90-minute cycles. That's why if you sleep for seven and half hours and wake up, you feel fresher, as you've finished that 'cycle' and your body finds it easier to wake up. If you wake up after 10 hours, you're mid-way through a cycle, which is why you feel tired, groggy and need a 'kick' just to get going the next morning.

Given that it is an essential way of resting, recharging and nourishing both your body and mind, sustained, unbroken sleep and dreaming are a part of our lifestyles that determine the quality of our lives and our health.

If you're living in a state of high performance, such as studying, training, working or are a full-time parent, then sleep should be a conscious act, not something that just happens. You have the power to take care of specific factors to make sure you're tired when you decide to sleep. This includes eating the right food at the right times, taking certain supplements and minimising the use of technology that upsets your body's melatonin production.

Three ways to diet-hack your sleep

1. **Fill up on fat:** After reading David Asprey's *The Bullet Proof Diet* and then testing out the effects of medium chain triglycerides oil (MCT) on my body and brain, I decided to use some version of MCT (from food or oils) throughout the day. I've not only noticed an improvement in my sleep quality, but my overall energy and brain 'clearness' throughout the day have improved.

> **'Fat is a long burning fuel for your mind and body'**
>
> **DAVID ASPREY.**

The shortest-length fats of MCT oil are converted into ketones that are immediately used as fuel for your brain, and MCT oil can also help burn body fat while you sleep. I've noticed that I think faster and more clearly the next morning if I've had MCT oil the night before.

I have also found that having slow-release complex carbohydrates such as oats before bed also helps me sleep better. This is because in this case, you're giving your body some glucose while you sleep as opposed to ketones from MCT. Both work great, and I recommend experimenting with both and see what works best for you.

Note: If you're not used to MCT oil, start slowly and make sure to mix it with some other component. I normally use whey or vegan rice protein. Too much MCT without your body being used to it can lead to a mild stomach upset.

2. **The power of protein:** Our bodies use protein for muscle repair and immune function. In the training section, I have discussed how you tear down fibres while you train. It's actually your diet and sleep that repair these fibres.

   The muscle repair occurs at night during your deep REM sleep, for which you require raw materials (amino acids) to help heal and grow new tissues. I recommend consuming a combination of a scoop of good-quality whey or vegan protein with a tablespoon of MCT oil 30 minutes before bed.

   Too much protein can raise the alertness chemical in the brain called orexin, which can disrupt your sleep. Therefore, it's important not to have 'too much' protein before bed.

For years, I used to have two chicken breasts before bed thinking that it would 'help me repair', not realizing that it was massively disrupting my quality of sleep. I scaled back 60g of protein to 25g of protein with 10–15g of fat or 20g of complex carbs and my sleep has never been better.

3. **Carbs before bed:** As mentioned above, some slow-release carbohydrates such as oats are a part of a great sleep hack. Your brain uses a lot of energy while you're asleep. One efficient form of brain energy comes from the sugar that is stored in the liver, called liver glycogen. Your brain taps your liver glycogen before hitting the stored sugar in your muscles (muscle glycogen). Therefore, having a little carbohydrate before bed can help your brain function better and allow you to relax and get into a deeper sleep.

   As mentioned in Nathaniel Altman's *The Honey Prescription*, a small amount of raw honey has a similar effect on relaxing your body before bed. Furthermore, combining honey with some MCT oil will not throw you out of the fat-burning mode, as the shortest-length MCT derived from a supplement produces ketones even in the presence of carbohydrates. Thus, you can stay in the mild state of ketosis even while sleeping. I found taking both slow-release carbohydrates like oats and honey in the combined form or by themselves to work great. Personally, I find oats help me sleep better, but I have several clients who prefer not to eat 'real food' before bed and find that the texture of honey works amazingly well for them.

How to supplement-hack your sleep

For some, using the food tricks and eliminating caffeine and stimulants closer to bed time is enough to get a great night's sleep. However, if you find yourself really needing a supercharge, there are some supplements that will work wonders for you by either helping you fall asleep or keeping you in a deeper sleep.

Always check your supplements to verify their compatibility with medications that you may be taking, as some vitamins and minerals have been known to reduce the effect of some medications, such as birth control pills. There are a number of great herbs and supplements that can help you get a great night's sleep. Here are some that I've found support me the best and that don't leave me feeling groggy in the morning.

Getting a great night's sleep is great, but if you wake up feeling foggy, it defeats the purpose.

1. Zinc

Zinc is an important supplement for male and female fertility and thereby for libido, as zinc deficiency can lead to lower testosterone levels. Both men and women need balanced testosterone levels for optimal hormonal support. Zinc can support testosterone production by putting you into a deeper sleep, which also improves recovery dramatically for athletes, as zinc is one of the first minerals to get depleted in gym-goers and athletes.

Dosage: *It is normally best taken at a dosage of 25mg per day with magnesium (see below) and vitamin B6 (ZMA) – about 30 minutes before bed on an empty stomach.*

2. Magnesium

Nowadays, nearly everyone is magnesium deficient. Refined/processed foods are stripped off their mineral, vitamin and fibre content. These are anti-nutrient foods because they actually steal magnesium in order to be metabolised. When consumed, if not supplemented with magnesium, we become increasingly deficient.

Are you tense and tight or crave chocolate? Anything that

makes you tense or tight could be potentially due to a magnesium deficiency, which is one reason why you may crave chocolate at night-time or when stressed. Chocolate is one of the highest food sources of magnesium. The case of consuming chocolate is a catch twenty-two though. Even though it has magnesium, chocolate also has sugar. Every molecule of sugar you consume pulls over 50 times the amount of magnesium out of the body.

Dosage *Try taking 600–800mg a day 30 minutes before bed. However, be careful, as too much too soon can give you a stomach upset. When you get the correct dosage, due to its mild affect on your central nervous system, you can find that you are much more relaxed going to bed.*

3. GABA

An inhibitory neurotransmitter, your brain uses GABA to shut itself down. It can dramatically calm you down when taken on an empty stomach. I normally take it 60 minutes after my meal. GABA is great at bed time, but can also be used during the day if you're highly stressed or dealing with anxiety.

Dosage: *Start with 500mg before bed. This dosage can*

go as high as 2,500mg (incrementing the dose). GABA has also been shown to raise human growth hormone (HGH) in the higher end of dosage (discussed below).

4. L-Tryptophan

Also sold as 5HTP, L-tryptophan is normally talked about after Christmas or thanksgiving dinner, as turkey is particularly high in this amino acid. L-tryptophan can allow your brain to release serotonin (one of our brains happy hormones), which can help you unwind before bed.

Dosage: *Start with 500mg a night.*

I've always been a massive fan of the ZMA, GABA and 5HTP combination, which always allows my body and brain to unwind at the right time, get into a deeper sleep and does not leave me groggy in the morning. There is one other great supplement that can be included for shorter periods of time, especially for the first few weeks of any new program in order to get your body into a good sleeping routine. That supplement is melatonin.

5. Melatonin

It is a potent hormone and antioxidant that your body is supposed to produce on its own if you get natural darkness (from the sun going down each day) and enough sleep. When I struggled with sleep in my mid twenties, I was getting neither, and a lot of people with sleep issues are the same. There is a risk of your body stopping the production of melatonin if you supplement with it, so I only recommend using it for short periods, not more than 4 weeks at a time, and then taking at least four to eight weeks off. Your body naturally regulates its production of hormones based on how much of those hormones are present in the body. Therefore, if you supplement with melatonin, your body will naturally produce less melatonin.

Dosage *Melatonin supplements can range from 300–3,000mg. I tend to stay on the lower end with 300–500mg if I use it for an extended period (4 weeks) or use the high end 3,000 mg for 2 or 3 days if I need to recover from jet lag. Keep this as a tool in your arsenal, but don't have it as a staple as with ZMA, GABA and 5HTP.*

Human growth hormone (HGH) and sleep

During sleep, your body naturally secretes HGH, which maintains your organs and tissues. Training and using the correct supplements can boost HGH dramatically, but sleep is another crucial factor responsible for maintaining optimal levels. As you get older, your natural level of HGH secretion drops. Therefore, using hacks, supplements, foods and sleep can give you all the benefits – lower body fat, more muscle, increased energy and anti-aging to name a few. If you want to remain full of energy, in a great physical condition and youthful, keeping your HGH high is critical. All the supplements mentioned above can dramatically increase natural HGH while you sleep.

How to avoid the night time second wind

There is a window from 10:45–11:00pm when most people naturally get tired. This window differs a little, based on each person or the current season, but it falls in with the general circadian cycle mentioned above. If you don't go to sleep then and choose to stay awake, you'll get a cortisol driven 'second wind' that can keep you awake until 2:00 or 3:00am.

This happened to me for years! If I missed my 11:00pm window by 15 or 20 minutes, I would get this incredible second wind, which was amazing when I was eighteen or nineteen and going out to clubs, but terrible when I was in my mid-twenties and had to be up for work at 6:00am.

If you can stick as close as you can to the circadian cycle and get to bed before 11:00pm, you will wake up feeling more rested than if you get the same amount of sleep starting later. I know it's hard for some people, especially if you work night shifts, as your circadian cycle is massively disrupted. But I recommend experimenting with this trick for a week or two.

Try going to bed at 12:00am, allowing for 30 minutes of unwind time beforehand, and getting up at 8:00am. The following week, try going to bed at 11:00pm and getting up at 7:00am and monitor how much better you feel when you do the latter. It seemed crazy to me initially. I thought seven-and–a-half hours sleep is seven-and-a-half hours regardless of when you get it, but the results were very different when put into practice. It's also great to know about this second wind as you can choose to avoid it or take advantage of it – some of my best writing and ideas have come to me during this second wind. Just be sure you don't have an early start the next morning.

Switch off your brain

The problem usually begins before bedtime. You may feel unable to switch off from feelings of stress, tension and anxiety. One thing that has supported me massively is writing down all of tomorrow's task before I get into my night-time routine. For months, I found myself thinking about what I had to do the next day, and it felt like my brain was going into an overdrive to solve all of life's problems at midnight! Writing down everything I need to do the following day helps my brain unwind, safe in the knowledge that I won't forget my most important tasks.

When you get right down to it, food is one of the most important variables that makes an impact on your energy levels and body composition. The second most important variable – which is probably just as important as exercise if not more – is sleep. You don't need to necessarily use all the tools, tips and supplements mentioned above, but having knowledge of them can make a massive difference in your quality of life and in finding out what works best for you and your body. By changing what you use, eat and do before bed can give you an edge in all other aspects of your life.

CHAPTER 4
ALCOHOL AND HYDRATION

ALCOHOL

I have a little bit of a love and hate relationship with alcohol. I love nothing more than a glass or two of wine with a meal, but I hate the feeling that comes with going over that amount. My goal here isn't to say alcohol is good or bad. It's more to give you an idea of what's happening to your body when you consume it and then let you decide if you should or shouldn't factor it into your plan each week.

Why alcohol can halt your progress

Alcohol is metabolized by the liver and thus drastically affects your blood sugar balance, particularly when consumed on an empty stomach – this is why you are 'starving' after you have had five or six drinks.

Drinking alcohol, particularly those drinks with added sugar, results in a rapid rise in blood sugar. This causes your pancreas to release insulin in an attempt to balance your blood sugar. Insulin circulates, does what it's supposed to do and then leaves you mildly hypoglycaemic (low blood sugar), making sure you are excessively hungry after several drinks. Therefore, on top of adding extra calories to your daily intake and dehydrating you, your blood sugar levels also get negatively affected. Thus, the next logical question is: 'Does having alcohol with food minimize its effects?' Not quite, I'm afraid.

Alcohol also works as a 'displacing agent', meaning when you consume alcohol with meals, it serves as a blocking agent, prohibiting the absorption of several vitamins and minerals.

Alcohol, fat loss and muscle building

Now that I've explained how alcohol affects your body, let's take a look at how it affects fat loss and muscle gain.

On one side, your body will not burn body fat or build lean muscle tissue while it's detoxifying itself of alcohol. However, on the other side, alcohol moves straight to the front of the queue as your primary energy source, which your body will burn through it as its 'go to' energy source while it's in your system.

Your body using alcohol as its main energy source is a lot like your car trying to run on water – it will just break down shortly after you get going. Have you ever gone for a run or a gym session the day after you have had four or five alcoholic drinks, to try and 'sweat' the alcohol out? And while working out, have you felt like it was coming out through your pores as you trained?

That being said, alcohol is one of the first things that I re-introduce in my programs once people hit their target weight or physique. This is because small amounts of alcohol, two or three glasses of wine on a Saturday night for example, will go straight to the front of the queue to be used as energy. So, if you train the following day, your body can potentially burn straight through any alcohol you drink.

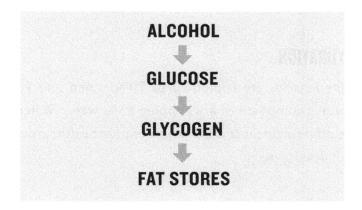

ALCOHOL
⬇
GLUCOSE
⬇
GLYCOGEN
⬇
FAT STORES

Further, irrespective of the above-mentioned negative effects of alcohol, the feeling of relaxation you get with a small amount of alcohol can do wonders for stress levels in certain people.

How to use: I recommend limiting alcohol until you get to your target weight or physique, then re-introduce it once or twice a week.

Tip: There are roughly 64 calories in a shot of clear alcohol, Vodka and Bacardi for example, and 82 calories in a glass of white wine. Beer has between 200 and 300 calories per pint. If you want to keep your calories on the lower side, limit your alcohol consumption to white wine and clear alcohol and save yourself a fortune in calories.

Comparison:s

3 pints of beer: 600–900kcal
3 glasses of white wine: 246kcal
3 glasses of vodka and diet mixer: 192kcal

HYDRATION

Your muscles are composed of 70% water, and your brain is composed of a whopping 95% water. Water is also the single most critical nutrient for health, growth and development.

A 2% drop in body water can cause a small yet critical shrinkage of the brain, which can impair coordination and massively decrease concentration. Dehydration can also reduce endurance, decrease strength, cause cramping and slow-down muscular response.

How much water do I need?

There is no 'one size fits all' to this question, but the general recommendation is two to three litres per day for women and three to four litres per day for men.

Of course, there are a lot of external factors that may require you to increase this amount. If you train regularly or live in hot weather conditions, your hydration requirement may go up.

For example, I train four or five times per week, so I normally drink around four litres per day.

Let your pee be your guide!

Your pee is normally your best indicator of your hydration level.

If it is clear, you're normally adequately hydrated. If it is light yellow and has an odour, you're one or two steps away from dehydration (light yellow with no smell can come from supplementing with too much vitamin B or a very high-dosed multi vitamin). If it is dark yellow and has an intense odour, you're probably dehydrated and not performing at your optimal level.

How to drink more water?

The key to drinking more water can be as simple as always carrying a water bottle with you. Leave it at your desk at work or beside you on the couch at home. If it's there and you see it, it will serve as an automatic subconscious reminder to drink more and stay hydrated. This has worked great for me, and I haven't left home without a two-litre water bottle in about five years.

CHAPTER 5
TRAINING

I remember getting a gym membership from my mum and dad for my sixteenth birthday and being extremely excited for my new fitness journey. I had been lifting weights, doing push-ups and pull ups at home and now that I was in the gym, I thought it was only a matter of months before I looked like one of the models from the magazines. Turns out, it doesn't really work that way.

One of the most disheartening things you may face when trying to get in shape, whatever that looks like for you, is putting in all the hard work and still not seeing the results. You eat what you think is good food, use supplements that you heard are good for losing fat or building muscle, and on top of that, you train every day and you still don't see the changes you want to see.

This can be incredibly frustrating. I remember how disheartened I felt after my first six months in the gym.

I must have made every training and nutrition mistake you can think of – I nearly quit a hundred times. This entire book is written on the premise that if I had read it when I started, I would have cut my learning curve by years.

When I first began training, I found the nutrition tricky but do-able. Supplements were a minefield, but when I indeed analysed this area, I found that there are only a few that you actually need. However, training was a different monster. I grew up with the mantra: 'The more effort you put in, the more you get out'. Therefore, to me, it sounded obvious that if I trained three hours a day, I'd get three times the results. However, training doesn't really work like that.

A funny thing happened when I started to cut my workouts from three hours to two hours and then to one hour – which is the most time I'll dedicate to workouts now – my body composition began to change, and I started to look better!

To me, it defied all logic – surely three hours is better than one, right? It turns out, your body is a complicated machine and like all machines, if you overwork and put too much strain on it, it can break down. That's what happened in my case. To physically change your body, I've found the optimal time to train is between 40 and 60 minutes a day, three to five times per week. That's not to say that you can't do great things by dedicating more or less than that, but I've found this to be the most optimal time in terms of physical results.

The analogy I like to make for getting in great shape is that of pushing a large and heavy wheel up a hill – it takes a lot of physical and mental effort to get the wheel moving initially, but once you create a bit of momentum, it becomes much easier. Keeping this analogy in mind, once you actually get the wheel to the top of the hill, it takes much less effort to just hold it there. Getting into the shape you want is similar. The beginning is hard, but once you get moving, create momentum along the way and begin to see changes, it becomes much easier. After you hit your target weight, body fat level or look, it becomes easier to sustain, provided you continue to use the blueprint that helped you get there in the first place – meal timings, making better food choices, exercising for tension and intensity, etc.

The real key is to make sure you overlap your goals with your training program. The truth is there is no single best training program – if there were just one, everyone would have followed it, and all the other training programs would have become obsolete. However, from my 17 years of training experience and having worked with thousands of people, I can say that there are certain systems, styles and programs that work great for body composition, which I'll discuss below.

What's the best kind of training?

There are numerous different training systems and styles that can work great for people, but I've found that in order to build a leaner, more muscular or toned physique, there's one thing that you need to do above all else – tear muscle fibres by creating tension on the muscle.

Burn fat while you watch TV

Tension-style training elicits a significant tear in muscle fibres, which can give a substantial boost to your metabolism. You burn more calories through such training. Have you ever read about how weight training allows you to burn calories while you watch your favourite TV show? Here's how.

When you weight train or work for resistance in general, using body weight, dumbbells, bands or barbells, etc., you tear more muscle fibres. These fibres need repairing after every workout, for which they use calories from the food and amino acids from protein.

Instead of those calories adding inches to your waistline, training effectively gives them another job to do – repair from the workout. In order for your muscles to repair, your metabolism has to increase, lending itself to burning more calories while you rest. Tension-style training and HIIT are great systems for 'getting a better bang for your buck', because you do less to get more. Depending on the program you are following, those torn muscle fibres could be repairing for up to 72 hours *after* the workout. Therefore, the food you eat goes towards repair and not into fat storage.

Tension-style training

Tension-style training means keeping the muscle you are working under optimal tension throughout the duration of the movement, i.e. two seconds on the way down, 1 second hold at the bottom or top and two seconds on the way up (2:1:2).

Have you ever done 10 repetitions of an exercise where you never really feel the muscle you were supposed to work, but just did the exercise 10 times because that's what was on your program or plan? The key to changing body composition, increasing metabolism and building a leaner body is to create tension on the muscle for every single rep. From the several variations of tension-style training, my favourite is the 2:1:2 systems, combined with focusing on the muscle you are trying to work – a mind–muscle connection. This style of training combined with the right program can change your body composition very quickly when combined with the right nutritional and supplement strategy.

Eccentric vs concentric

Just to expand on 2:1:2, you could use the term 'eccentric' (negative portion of the rep) and 'concentric' (positive portion of the rep) to better understand it. Every exercise below focuses on 2:1:2. Therefore, whether it's a dumbbell bench press or a leg press, you will lower the weight for two seconds, hold and pause for one second on the bottom or top of movement and raise the weight for two seconds.

You can vary this tempo for extra tension, replacing two seconds with four seconds for example, on the lowering or raising of each rep. The take-home message is that it's not about moving the weight from A to B – the aim is to create optimal tension for the duration of the movement and actually 'feel' the muscle you are working as a mind–muscle connection.

Mind-muscle connection

Have you ever just moved a weight from A to B, not really feeling any particular muscle? You know it hurts and you are clearly working out, but you can't really pinpoint what muscle you worked? That's from a lack of mind–muscle connection.

It's exactly as it sounds. You want your mind connected to the muscle you are working. For example, if you are doing a dumbbell bent over row, you want to feel your back on each rep. However, the closest muscles to your grip are your forearms and bicep. Therefore, normally those muscles can kick in and fatigue before you have even worked your back. This is where the 2:1:2 system really shines, because you are not moving weight from A to B; you are moving a weight with perfect form, creating optimal tension on the muscle you are trying to work (back in this case) from A to B. This way, you can create more tension on the muscle without having to go 'super heavy', which increases your risk of injury and which will in turn massively reduce your progress.

I've followed this exact training program, and I can only lift 4kg or 5kg on side lateral raise for shoulders for example. If you are able to lift 25 kg with perfect form on this movement, you either have super human strength or you are swinging with momentum, meaning that you are not working the muscle for optimal tension. The best piece of gym advice that I have received was 'Leave your ego at the door'. I generally find women much better at this, but an added note for any men reading this: if you are trying to get a leaner, toned and more muscular physique, but feel you need to constantly out-lift your training partners with super heavy weight on a bench press or a barbell curl, it might be worth considering that you change your training partners.

Don't get me wrong, you still want to find a weight that is heavy enough so that you are failing at your given rep range. When I say I use 5kg on side lateral raises, that's physically the heaviest weight I can lift with perfect form creating optimal tension on the side deltoid (the muscle I'm working). You may need to use 10kg or 12kg to create the same tension. Just be careful not to swing the weight with momentum. With the exception of a system called 'cheat reps', where you use a slight momentum at the end of an exercise when you hit muscular failure, if you are doing it from your first rep, that's just bad form.

Building a mind-muscle connection with every body part doesn't happen overnight, and you will find it much harder to connect with certain exercises or body parts than with others. For example, it took me years to learn to 'feel' my legs when I trained them. I would move a weight from A to B, and my legs never really responded. It wasn't until I learnt about creating optimal muscular tension and started implementing it in my own training that they responded. Now they are probably my strongest body parts. So if you struggle to feel your glutes, chest or biceps, remember that I was there too, but with the right system, you can turn your weakest body part into the strongest.

Form: it's not about the weight, it's about how you move the weight.

Creating optimal tension and feeling the muscle you are trying to work is indeed the secret to a better body composition. However, you also need to do it right. When you hear people talking about their 'form', it's actually just the way you do the movement. If you do a barbell bent over row with a curved back, that's considered 'bad form', which basically means that you're not performing the movement the correct way. As you are not swinging the weight from A to B, the beauty of tension training and 2:1:2 systems means you can focus on creating the tension on every single rep. As mentioned above, I'm not saying to go super light. You want to pick a weight that enables you to perform the movements within the perfect form and fail at the given rep range. This leads to one of my most frequently asked questions: 'How do I pick the right weight?'

How to pick the right weight

For example, if you're doing your 'push' workout in the 10-rep range on Monday, you're moving a weight in the 2:1:2 system on an incline dumbbell press and could have easily completed 12, 13 or 14 reps with that weight, that particular weight is too light and you need to go heavier.

Conversely, if you're aiming for 10 reps and fail at five or six reps, the weight is too heavy and you need to reduce it.

The key is keeping track of the weight you used and always trying to fail at your given rep range, which is 10 reps in this program.

Sometimes, you will get tired and fail before the 10 reps on your last set. There are two systems that I would like to include here. One is a 'drop set' and the other is a 'rest pause' technique.

For example, if you are doing three sets of 10 reps on incline dumbbell press with 20kg and on your third set, you fail at seven reps, you can either drop the weight by 25% to 15kg and finish your last three reps (this is called a drop set), or you can go back to your starting position, rest for 5 or 10 seconds and finish your three reps with the 20 kg (this is called a rest pause). Both systems work incredibly well and can be used interchangeably. My advice would be to use a rest pause on busier gym days, so that you don't lose your bench or need extra sets of dumbbells and use drop sets when training at home or on quieter gym days.

What's the best cardio?

Losing body fat and getting into your best possible shape may require at least some aerobic activity. The range of aerobic methods and the different systems available in cardio are many – enough to cause confusion for the most dedicated fitness enthusiasts.

Aerobic activity by its very nature requires fat to be used as a primary fuel source, with carbohydrates and protein being used to a smaller extent. Therefore, if fat loss is your primary goal, some degree of aerobic work will help you a lot.

Aerobic activities can include the following:

• Running

- Walking

- Cycling

- Swimming

- Bodyweight HIITs

- Resistance HIIT

There is no 'one best cardio' or aerobic activity. The key is to find the one you enjoy the most, which your body responds to, normally by reducing body fat and then using that as your primary source of cardio. If you hate to run, try swimming or cycling. If you love team sports, join a sports club and get your cardio that way.

Try HIIT cardio for faster fat loss

The two main types of cardio are low-intensity steady state cardio (LISS) and high-intensity interval training (HIIT). Both are great and both work very well.

Low intensity steady state (LISS) is exactly as it sounds – it's low in intensity. For example, a 15-minute steady pace walk, jog or cycle where you are at or above 70% of your max heart rate.

Note: 70% of your max heart rate is your 'fat-burning zone' – to calculate your max heart rate, subtract your *age from 220. For example, if you are 28, it would be 220 minus 28, which is 192.*

LISS is a good tool if your diet is clean – your carbs are low and you're eating regular meals throughout the day alongside your weight-training program. But I've found that you do need to do longer spells of LISS, normally 15–20 minutes or more to see any noticeable changes.

HIIT on the other hand is 'sprint training'. Its benefits are that it's quick (five to ten minutes normally), burns through more glycogen (stored carbohydrates) and gives you a great feeling of accomplishment upon finish. Its negatives are that it's difficult. And when done correctly, very difficult!

There are hundreds of ways to incorporate HIIT into your program (Tabata, 20:40 sprints, outdoor 20 –100m sprinting), but my favourite method is 10 minutes of 30:30 HIIT.

For 30:30 HIIT, you have 30 seconds 'on' or sprint time and 30 seconds 'off' for rest or recovery time. This can be done on a bike, treadmill, with battle ropes or bodyweight movements (spider push-ups/burpee, etc.). The key is to go as hard as possible for 30 seconds and then completely rest or recover for the next 30 seconds.

Time your HIIT for faster fat loss

Depleting your glycogen levels by doing your weight training first and your cardio after could potentially allow you to tap into fat stores more effectively. Of course, as long as you are doing your cardio or getting your heart rate up alongside all the other tips mentioned in this book, you will burn body fat. This is just a quick tip that could potentially allow you to do it faster.

To explain this further, check out the two hypothetical scenarios given below: This applies to both genders so feel free to switch John's name for Jane's below if you prefer.

Scenario 1

John Smith trains five days every week for 60 minutes on the cross trainer. He had white pasta and chicken in his last meal. After 20 or 30 minutes on the cross trainer, John finally depletes his glucose (from his pasta meal) and is now using glycogen as his energy source. Another 30 minutes pass, and John is still using glycogen as his energy source. He leaves his workout happy that he got to the gym. Two months later, after going to the gym five days a week, John hasn't lost any body fat, built any muscle or changed at all, and quits. Does this sound familiar?

Scenario 2

Jane Smith trains four days every week for 60 minutes. She does tension-style weight training for 45 minutes and finishes with 10 minutes of high-intensity cardio at the end of every workout. Her pre-workout meal was chicken or fish, mixed vegetables and one tablespoon of almond butter or 150g of sweet potato. As she is focused on tension during her weight training, she is burning through all the glucose in her body at a pretty rapid rate – she's not even half way through her workout, and is now very likely to be tapping into her stored carbohydrates (glycogen).

Twenty minutes later, her glycogen is nearly completely depleted and she is now using fat as her primary fuel source. She finishes her workout with 10 minutes of HIIT. Two months later, Jane is leaner, fitter, slimmer, more toned, feels better and continues to train for the rest of the year.

Now, ask yourself which scenario you would.

Remember, progress is addictive: I don't know a person in the world who could continue a workout regime with absolutely no progress. So arm yourself with knowledge and get better results in less time.

THE TRAINING PROGRAM

Push, pull, legs

There are hundreds of training programs that work fantastically well. However, having worked with thousands of clients all over the world, one of my favourite systems has to be the 'Push, pull, legs' split, as it allows you to train every body part at least once per week or twice per week if you're training five or six days.

'Push, pull, legs' is the name of the training split for the movement patterns of that specific muscle group. 'Push' refers to all the movements where you use muscles that push the weight away from your body as their primary movement pattern – chest, shoulders and triceps. In 'pull', all the exercise is geared at pulling the weight toward your body as the muscles' primary movement patterns – back, rear delts and biceps. 'Legs' refers to lower body-focused leg training.

How to lay-out your training week

First, I would decide on how many days a week you are committed to training and then lay out your week around your schedule and lifestyle. I find that three days a week works great for beginners and four to five days a week for intermediate and advanced training. I like push, pull, legs, push, pull for my own five-day training split, but you need to find what works best for you. It's similar to the best time of the day to train – the best time is whenever it fits best into your schedule. If you only have an hour in the morning before work or at lunchtime, then that's the best time. If you use training as your 'de-stress' from work, then evening may be best for you. Laying out your week is similar. Your lifestyle might lend itself to training Monday to Friday, taking the weekends off. Others will be better with 'day on, day off', and those who can only train three days with Monday, Wednesday and Friday. Find the day and time that works best for your lifestyle and then adjust your schedule accordingly. Make training a priority, but try to fit it around your lifestyle and not the other way around.

Training program details

Exercise: The name of the exercise you will perform.

Reps: The number of repetitions you will do, the number of times you will perform the movements. For example, if you do the movement 10 times, that's 10 reps.

Sets: The number of sets is the number of 'rounds' you do. For example, if you do 3 sets of 10 reps, you perform 10 reps of the exercise with a 2:1:2 tempo and then rest for 60 seconds. Repeat for your second and third set.

Rest: The amount of time you rest in between sets.

Tension: All the reps are at a tension of 2:1:2. Two seconds on the positive (the upward motion), one second squeeze (at the top or bottom depending on the exercise) and two seconds on the negative (the downward motion).

Cardio: All the cardio in this program is based on HIIT. HIIT burns more calories, takes less time and works incredibly well to elevate metabolism while burning fat when incorporated into a tension styled program. I personally like using the rowing machine or a stationary bike, but HIIT can be done on any cardio machine.

HIIT: For HIIT training, set a level that you can sprint as fast as you can for 30 seconds. After 30 seconds, reduce the level to a very easy pace and recover for these seconds. Repeat this process 10 times for a total of 10 minutes.

Timing of each workout

Each workout should take between 40–60 minutes. This program is about quality over quantity. Therefore, bring a stopwatch to time your rest periods, train intensely while in the gym and get out within 60 minutes, so that you don't start to burn through any hard-earned muscle or overstress your central nervous system.

Track your weight

As the weeks progress, your body will be getting stronger in each exercise. Therefore, increase the weight every week (if needed) so that you fail at 10 repetitions during each workout.

For example, if you're lifting 10kg on incline dumbbell press, you may need to increase this to 12.5kg after one or two weeks as your muscles get stronger.

TRAINING PROGRAM VIDEOS

The entire training program is present below, but if you go to *www.briankeanefitness.com* you can download the videos that wgo through the entire workout and on how to perform each move correctly.

TRAINING PROGRAM TABLE

PUSH WORKOUT	
CHEST DUMBBELL PRESS	10 reps 3 sets 60 second rest 2:1:2 tempo
CHEST DUMBBELL FLYE	10 reps 3 sets 60 second rest 2:1:2 tempo
MILITARY BARBELL PRESS	10 reps 3 sets 60 second rest 2:1:2 tempo
SIDE LATERAL DUMBBELL RAISE	10 reps 3 sets 60 second rest 2:1:2 tempo
TRICEPS E-Z BAR LYING EXTENSION	10 reps 2 sets 60 second rest 2:1:2 tempo

TRICEPS ROPE EXTENSION

10 reps
2 sets
60 second rest
2:1:2 tempo

IO MINUTES OF 30:30 BIKE

PULL WORKOUT

BARBELL BENT OVER ROW

10 reps
3 sets
60 second rest
2:1:2 tempo

LAT PULL DOWN

10 reps
3 sets
60 second rest
2:1:2 tempo

REAR DELT DUMBBELL RAISE

10 reps
2 sets
60 second rest
2:1:2 tempo

ROPE REAR DELT FACE PULL

10 reps
2 sets
60 second rest
2:1:2 tempo

BARBELL BICEP CURL

10 reps

3 sets

60 second rest

2:1:2 tempo

DUMBBELL TWIST BICEP CURL

10 reps

3 sets

60 second rest

2:1:2 tempo

10 MINUTES OF 30:30 BIKE

LEGS WORKOUT

BARBELL SQUAT

10 reps

3 sets

60 second rest

2:1:2 tempo

DUMBBELL STANDING LUNGE

10 reps

3 sets

60 second rest

2:1:2 tempo

LEG PRESS

10 reps

3 sets

60 second rest

2:1:2 tempo

LEG EXTENSION

10 reps

3 sets

60 second rest

2:1:2 tempo

BARBELL GLUTE BRIDGE

10 reps

3 sets

60 second rest

2:1:2 tempo

STIFF-LEGGED DUMBBELL DEAD-LIFT

10 reps

2 sets

60 second rest

2:1:2 tempo

HAMSTRING CURL

10 reps

2 sets

60 second rest

2:1:2 tempo

SEATED CALF RAISE

20 reps

1 sets

2:1:2 tempo

NO CARDIO

SECTION 2
MINDSET

CHAPTER 6
CREATING HABITS

Now that you have knowledge on how to use nutrition, training and supplementation to increase your energy and get into a better shape, it's key to build a mindset that not only allows you to get what you want in the first place, but also possess all the tools required to sustain it.

For years, I would get very close to all the things I wanted in life. I'd be right on the verge of the body I wanted, leaving my job to start my own business or within touching distance of some other goal, and I would inevitably self-sabotage myself. Consciously or subconsciously, most of us have done it at some stage. We convince ourselves that it's not practical to leave a job or spend an hour a day in the gym when we have children, a full-time job and a mortgage to pay. We let the fear creep in, and this fear, if left unchecked, can paralyze us. For years, I would let fear creep in, and before I would know, I would be back to square one. This section of the book is designed to help bulletproof your mind so that you don't become your own worst enemy on the path to getting what you want. As Buddha once said, 'Don't let your own worst enemy live between your two ears.' The section covers everything from creating habits and dealing with anxiety, worry and stress to practical life tips that I read every morning in the hopes of passing them onto my daughter someday.

The first audio book I ever listened to was *The Power of Habit* by Charles Duhigg, which changed the way I looked at everything I did in my life.

At the time, I was working as a primary school teacher in West London and had picked up quite a few bad habits: I would come home after work every day, sit in the same chair, watch the same game show and have two or three chocolate bars as I numbed out to TV. I was starting to lose my shape and my energy levels plummeted. I had created a bad habit.

Creating positive habits and breaking negative ones

Charles Duhigg talks about the 'routine – cue – reward'

system of habits. In order to change a habit, you need to change one of the components of this system. The routine is the actual situation or 'trigger' – for me, the routine was coming home every day after work. The cue is what you do next, i.e. getting two or three bars from the cupboard and sitting in the same seat watching the same show. And the reward is serotonin release, the 'happy hormone' your brain releases from the chocolate.

As soon as I realized this was affecting me negatively, I put plans in place to change one of the components. For me, the routine of coming home from work was always going to be the same, so I changed the cue. Instead of reaching for chocolate bars in the cupboard, I left a pre-packed gym bag beside the front door. I would come home (routine), pick up my gym bag (new cue) and the reward came via the serotonin release from exercise.

Becoming self-aware of your negative behaviour, patterns and habits isn't always that easy to recognize. That's why reading certain books is crucial, as they can 'point' things out in a way that we may have missed or failed to see.

I tried and lived my life by internalizing that there are only three ways to look at most of the things in your life: 1) the things you know; 2) the things you don't know; and 3) the things you don't know you don't know.

I used and still use books, podcasts and following the right people on social media to bridge the gap between all three.

The story of the boy and the tree

The *Power of Habit* made me understand that I was living in a pattern without even realizing it. The book bridged that gap and put me in a much more positive place mentally and physically. Some habits are harder to change than others.

I remember hearing a story in my early twenties that I never truly forgot. It was about a wise teacher and his student. Both were taking a stroll through a forest when the teacher stops before a tiny tree and turns to his student 'Pull up that sapling', pointing to a sprout newly emerging from the earth. The youngster pulls it up easily with his fingers. 'Now pull up that one', says the teacher to the boy, indicating a more established sapling that has grown to about knee-high length. With a little effort, the lad yanks the plant and it comes off, uprooted. 'And now, this one', says the teacher, nodding toward a more well-evolved evergreen that is as tall as the young pupil. With great effort, throwing all his weight and strength into the task, using sticks and stones, the pupil pries up the stubborn roots, getting the tree loose. 'Now', the wise one says, 'I'd like you to pull this one up.' The young boy follows the teacher's gaze and sees a mighty oak, so tall the boy can scarcely see the top. Knowing the struggle he'd just had pulling up a much smaller tree, he simply tells the teacher, 'I am sorry, but I can't.' The teacher exclaims, 'My son, you have just demonstrated the power that habits will have over your life! The older they are, the bigger they get, the deeper the roots grow, and the harder they are to uproot. Some get so big, with roots so deep, you might hesitate to try to uproot them.'

Smaller bad habits like the one I mentioned above are easy to change by understanding the 'routine – cue – reward' system – you just change one of those components and you can effectively change your habits. Some habits are harder to break than others, some have 'deeper roots' – for example, if you have never felt confident about the way you look or have been overweight your entire life, you're not going to do something and wake up lean and skinny or full of confidence overnight.

It's the deep-rooted habits that are more difficult to change. It's the small things every day that allow you to change these habits. I have worked with people who have been overweight their entire life who get frustrated when they're not lean in two weeks. If I said to you that I wanted to learn Spanish, but I wanted to be fluent in two weeks, what would you tell me? It's probably not possible, right? But what if I said I wanted to be fluent in six, twelve or eighteen months? Then it becomes a lot more realistic. Breaking bad habits is the same – you're not going to break a habit that you've had for five, ten or even twenty years in two weeks. But by taking the right steps, you could break it in six or twelve months and then be rid of it forever. Aristotle wrote, 'We are what we repeatedly do.'

Are you riding the horse of your habits and getting nowhere?

There's a great story in Darren Hardy's *The Compound Effect* about a man riding a horse, galloping fast. It appears that's he's going somewhere very important. A man standing along the roadside shouts, 'Where are you going?' The rider replies, 'I don't know. Ask the horse!'

Darren Hardy describes that this is the story of most people's lives – they're riding a horse of their habits, with no idea where they're headed. Psychological studies reveal that 95% of everything we feel, think, do and achieve is a result of a learned habit.

We do most things in life in autopilot. When was

the last time you thought about how you tied your shoelaces or how you brushed your teeth? If you're like me, you probably even put on the same shoe first (left one) every single day and don't even consciously realize you're doing it. Thinking about habits this way can indeed help you understand how important it is to create positive ones.

If you eat healthily, you've likely built healthy habits around food – what you put in your shopping basket or what you order in restaurants becomes automatic. The same thing happens if you eat unhealthily – you make different choices automatically.

How to make the right automatic choice

The key is educating yourself about what foods are good choices for your body and mind (see the nutrition section of this book) and then create habits accordingly, so that those food choices become automatic. The key to sticking to a good nutritional plan is finding or creating a plan that includes your preferences – foods you like, enjoy and that work into your lifestyle and schedule. If you can make your nutrition automatic, it becomes the way you eat and not a diet you're following. In other words, eating well becomes a habit.

With enough practice and repetition, any behaviour, good or bad becomes automatic over time. The key is having conscience thought and self-awareness about which habits are supporting you and which ones are destructive to your life. If your goal is to lose body fat, build more muscle or have more energy throughout the day, understand which habits you need to break or create in order to become that person. After that, it's about following the right habits on a consistent basis.

Even though we develop most of our habits unconsciously, by modelling our parents, responding to environmental or cultural associations, or creating coping mechanisms, we can consciously decide to change them. Reflect on how deeply your habits are rooted and then put the plan in place to create new positive ones in their place. Sometimes, it's as easy as making the decision and then using your 'why' to get you there.

CHAPTER 7
FIND YOUR WHY

The how means nothing until you find your why

Finding your why can be the ultimate difference between getting what you want and giving up before you even start. All of the 'hows' mean nothing until you find your 'why'.

My 'why' is my little girl, Holly. The day my daughter was born, there was a 'fire lit under me'. I was doing okay before that – I enjoyed my life, I was happy with what I was doing, but now it wasn't about me anymore – it was about us.

The reason my life took such a dramatic turn over the past few years is because things like my health now became more important to me. I was competing at the top level of my sport in competitive bodybuilding and travelling the world as a professional fitness model, but I was living a lifestyle that definitely wasn't focused on my health – weeks before shows, I couldn't hold a conversation with people due to my body being so calorie and food restricted.

I remember sitting in my living room on a cold autumn day, mapping out the shows for that coming year. Suddenly, a vision came into my mind, of Holly trying to play with me while I'm lying on a couch with no energy because I'm 'too tired' and her saying, 'What's wrong with Daddy, why won't he play with me?' That vision broke my heart and that was the day my path changed direction. I had a new 'why'.

If your why power (or desire) isn't great enough, it's likely that any goal will end up like most new-year resolutions – you will pursue the goal for two, three maybe even four weeks and then life will get in the way and you will slowly or gradually stop or quit. We've all done that.

I will give you 100 euros to walk across this plank

Think of it this way: If I were to put a 10-inch-wide, 30-foot-long plank on the ground and say, 'if you walk the length of the plank, I'll give you 100 euros, would you do it? Of course, it's easy money.

But what if I took the same plank and made a roof-top bridge between two 100-story buildings? Then that money would not look as desirable and you probably wouldn't even consider doing the task for a second. However, imagine if your child were on the opposite building, and the building were on fire, would you walk across the length of the plank to save him/her? You would be gone before you even thought about it.

Why is it that the first time you wouldn't cross the roof top plank, but the second time, you wouldn't even hesitate? The risks and the dangers are the same. What changed? Your 'why' changed, your reason for wanting to do it changed. When the reason is big enough and your why is strong enough, you will be willing to achieve your goal no matter what it takes.

I am fortunate enough to have an amazing life. I have what I call a 'non job' where my life and my job are one and the same. I have a healthy daughter whom I love more than anything in this world and an inner circle of friends and family who help me grow as a person. However, like everyone, there are days when 'I just don't feel like it'. Even the most successful people in the world (note: success is subjective to each person) have days when they struggle. The only difference between them and everyone else is they use their 'why' on those days.

I have a picture of Holly beside my bed and, on the mornings I don't want to get up at six o'clock, I look at that picture and remember my 'why'. I think to myself, 'if I don't get up, if I don't work, she doesn't eat'. That's extreme, but that's the difference it makes between getting up and getting dressed or hitting the snooze on my alarm. Finding your why, what drives you, can make the ultimate difference between getting and not getting everything you want in your life

How to find your why

'All of us, throughout our lives, have learned certain patterns of thinking and behaving to get ourselves out of pain and into pleasure'

TONY ROBBINS

We all experience emotions like frustration, anger or being overwhelmed and develop a strategy to end these feelings. Some people use food, some use sex, drugs or alcohol. Others use running, going to the gym or reading.

Sometimes your pain point can be your strongest why. The pain of envisioning my little girl upset because 'Daddy wouldn't play with her because he's too tired' is a pain that completely shifted my focus in life. My why is now to create and design a life where I have the time, money and health to truly be present before my daughter and influence her life in a positive way. Her journey is her journey, and I have no control over it, but I have control over how much I am present in this journey and how much influence, advice and guidance I can provide to help develop her character along the way.

Your why might be completely different from mine, and you might even have several 'whys'. It might be a comment or a jibe from a friend or a loved one that gives you that spark to get into great shape or a friend who called you stupid that led you to read more books (my why for indulging in reading).

'Your why needs to be greater than you'

ERIC THOMAS.

Pain and negativity can be powerful motivational tools and as long as they don't consume you, I think they're vital for achieving great things in life. Thus, on days when you're struggling and want to give up, recall the pain that made you get started and remember your why. Your why will keep you going on the days you want to give up. Use your why and go get what you want.

CHAPTER 8
STRESS

How can stress ruin your body and mind?

It's three o'clock in the morning and you're lying in bed. You have something immensely important or challenging to do the next day – a meeting at work, several lunches to make for the kids or an early morning workout that you can't miss.

You think to yourself, 'What if I don't hear my alarm and sleep in. I'll miss that meeting, my kids will starve or I won't get time for my workout and I'll be in bad mood all day'. Next thing you know, the alarm goes off and you were only asleep for a couple of hours.

You are incredibly tired but pull yourself out of the bed, get some coffee, tea or caffeinated drink, go to work, eat something sugary or stimulated to wake you up more, power through the day only to fall asleep in front of the TV for 20 minutes from pure exhaustion before everyone else gets home.

You wake from your short catnap, jump up, make dinner or go to the gym – finally catching your second wind. Then 11pm arrives, you settle down to bed only to find yourself staring at the ceiling for the second night in a row. Sounds familiar? This happens for two or three days in a row and then it hits you – a cold, flu or just a general feeling of being run down and being extra tired. Your energy is sapped, you find it even harder to get up in the morning and you are counting down to the weekend so you can sleep in. Looking at it, it's pretty easy to determine that this probably isn't the optimal way to get into a great shape and have more energy.

Nevertheless, this was my life pattern for nearly four years when I worked as a primary school teacher in London. I would lie awake in the bed on a Sunday night worrying that I would miss my alarm the next day and my whole week would be ruined.

Sleep, anxiety, worry and stress are something that have affected me a lot during my life. Thankfully, since understanding what was happening on a physiological and neurological level, realising that there was nothing actually wrong with me and that those feelings were pretty common has allowed me to find strategies to 'hack' that stress, worry or anxiety in my own life.

I'm not a physiologist or a clinical psychologist. I am just someone who was interested in finding out why I felt so anxious, worried and stressed all the time. As it had a direct impact on my health, energy and fitness and of those with whom I work, I always found myself fascinated by the psychology and neuroscience about what happens on a physiological level. Over a five-year period, I read and studied everything I could get my hands on to try to educate myself as to why I felt this way.

The section will talk about how stress, anxiety and worry can negatively affect your body's ability to get in shape. I hope it will help you as much as it helped me.

Understanding cortisol

Cortisol is your body's natural response to stress, and it can be a good or a bad thing depending on when it's released. Cortisol is a hormone released from the hypothalamus in your brain (a gland that connects your endocrine and nervous systems), pituitary gland (an endocrine gland at the base of the hypothalamus) and your adrenal gland (an endocrine gland on top of your kidneys).

All three of these glands work together as an axis while utilizing other hormones and precursors to make and release cortisol in times of stress. We can be pretty thankful for our body's ability to make cortisol because if you needed to run away from a sabre-toothed tiger thousands of years ago, you needed that instant energy that cortisol produces by engaging our fight, flight or flee response.

Just like any other hormone, there is a delicate range of how much our bodies can handle – too little or too much and things start going haywire. Too much stress in your life keeps the cortisol pumping and can have negative effects on your body, mind and physique. For anyone trying to stay healthy and look good, this can be a critical factor that you haven't thought of yet. Stress is the figurative 'death by a thousand cuts' – you can get everything right with your nutrition, training and supplementation, but if you are in a constant state of fight or flight, stress or anxiety, you are going to struggle to hit your own natural potential.

What causes stress and how to deal with it

Perhaps the best way to begin is by making a mental list of the sort of things that you find stressful. You would no doubt immediately come up with some obvious examples – a partner, family, friends who are always negative, or something more abstract, things like traffic jams, the gym at rush hour or work deadlines. You might even find things like 'not looking a certain way' or 'comparing yourself to others' as your main stressors; two areas I had issues with personally.

Thinking about these people, situations or events can trigger an automatic release of cortisol throughout our body. Has someone ever made you so mad that even the thought of them sent blood running through your veins? That's cortisol. Have you ever found your brain racing at 3:00am because you are worried about not waking up from your alarm – yeah, cortisol showing up. How about seeing that guy or girl that you find attractive who you just can't bring yourself to talk to?

That's cortisol again.

As I've mentioned, cortisol in short bursts can be incredibly beneficial. You actually release cortisol when you exercise, and it's needed for your body's ability to release glucose from the cells. However, chronic cortisol or stress can be detrimental to your physique, your health and your mindset. The next section is dedicated to understanding all the stressors that can secretly hinder your progress: anxiety, worry and some practical life tips that have supported me throughout my life in reducing cortisol and stress.

CHAPTER 9
ANXIETY

When I used to work as a primary school teacher in London, I remember regularly staring at the ceiling in my box room apartment with my head in my hands unable to sleep due to anxiety. Practically, I knew how ridiculous it was. I had a roof over my head, food in my stomach and a job to go to in the morning, but I still couldn't help the feeling that would well up inside of me. I would lie awake worrying if I was going to be able to pay my rent that month or about how my assessment at work would go the following week.

I actually felt like my heart was in my mouth, which would regularly lead to sleepless nights and continued for over four years of my stay in London. This of course eventually led to me consuming a lot of stimulated drinks or eating sugary food the following day to try and pick myself up. This cycle would ultimately keep me awake again the following night.

Every week, I would count down until Friday, so I could sleep in at the weekend and not set an alarm. Of course, the anxiety would subside every Friday evening, and I would stay awake until I was tired and then sleep right through the night. But alas, Saturday night would come and I would worry if I didn't sleep well that night, then my sleep pattern would be out of sync on the Sunday and I'd start the week off like I finished the previous one.

When I look back now, I see how ridiculous the whole thing was. But this pattern continued for months and months until I learnt that there was actually a legitimate physiological reason that I felt this way. I had anxiety.

I always thought anxiety meant that you didn't have your life together (regardless of what you may see, nobody has every area of their life together) and my only experience with anxiety was when work colleagues would get signed off work due to stress.

I didn't have enough self awareness to realise that it's something that all of us face at some time or another: for some people, it's chronic and affects them every single day, and the mere thought of something bad happening can set them off. For others, it can be chemically induced (too much caffeine, alcohol, drugs, etc.). Regardless, the more people I meet or clients I work with, the more I realise that everyone experiences anxiety in some way, shape or form.

> 'I've had a lot of worries in my life, most which never happened'
>
> **MARK TWAIN**

There are some serious cases of anxiety, and if you have suffered any major physical or mental trauma or have a hormonal imbalance, it would be probably best to consult your physician. However, I hope by sharing my own experiences and strategies, I will ultimately support you in managing any kind of day-to-day anxiety or worry that may be limiting you in any aspect of your own life.

What exactly is anxiety?

Anxiety is a complex emotional response that's similar to fear. Both anxiety and fear arise from similar brain processes and cause similar physiological and behavioural reactions: rapid heart rate, breathing disturbances and 'heart in mouth' feeling or the 'fight, flight or flee' response. The thing that's always made me curious about anxiety and fear (I regularly got them mixed up) is that fear is typically associated with a clear, present and identifiable threat, whereas anxiety occurs in the absence of an immediate threat.

Fear and anxiety are so closely related that we regularly confuse them. We feel fear when we are actually in trouble, like when someone overtakes a car on the opposite side of the road and is coming directly toward you. We feel anxiety when we have a sense of dread or discomfort, but at that moment, we are in no immediate danger.

Everyone experiences fear and anxiety. It's a part of everyday life and an evolutionary adaption: fear and anxiety probably kept your ancestors alive thousands of years ago – if you didn't feel those emotions, you were likely to be eaten by something higher in the food chain. However, all fear and anxiety do now is make us miserable and unhappy.

Have you ever had a roof over your head, food in the cupboards, a nine-to-five job and still worried about not having enough money in your bank account? I know I have.

Have you ever seen friends in loving relationships and think 'I'm never going to meet someone'? Yeah, I've been there too.

How about those times when you felt just 'off' for no reason other than not feeling right – you just felt on edge, but everything in your life was perfectly fine. This affected me for years until I better understood how certain food ingredients, (additives, flavourings etc.) of certain processed foods had a direct impact on my mood and anxiety levels. If you want to know more about this, take a look at the nutrition section of the book if you've not done so yet.

None of these feelings are fear, as you are in no immediate threat. This is anxiety.

Why your dog might be happier than you

Alongside cutting-out foods with those ingredients that sent my body into severe 'fight or flight' mode and made me edgy for days, the biggest thing that has supported me is knowing what was actually happening to my brain when I started to feel this way.

You're possibly familiar with the pre-frontal cortex – the 'thinking part' of the brain. It's what separates humans from other species – it enables us to use reason, create language and envision the future.

Have you ever wondered why your dog gets happy every single time they see you? Dogs and other animals haven't developed the part of the brain that allows them to picture the future, so when they see you, they are completely present every single time. They're not worried about when you will go again, whether they will get food that day or any other scenario that may or may not happen.

Although developing our pre-frontal cortex has allowed us to build civilisations and create things beyond our wildest dreams, the trade off is we can sometimes lack 'being present' – or being in the actual moment because we are thinking about the future. Nine out of ten times, it's normally worrying about something that hasn't even happened yet – work the next day, paying our bills, etc. This is normally the foundation of anxiety.

Fear is an immediate threat, whereas anxiety is thinking about a potential threat. There are cases where there is a genuine hormonal disruption and several of these people find western medicine great for their anxiety. However, for a lot of us, it's something we can control ourselves. I love the quote: 'Worrying is like a rocking chair, it gives you something to do but you never get anywhere'. As someone who would be fine for several days at a time and then get hit with a wave of anxiety like a brick to the head, there are a few things that have massively supported me. So, I'll share them below in the hopes that they support you.

Anxiety hacks and how to deal with it

1. **Recognise the source of your anxiety**
    'Find the source, fix the problem.' For some of us, it is as simple as cutting the source of anxiety. In my case, there were certain people in my life who just made me feel 'off'. I felt more insecure around them, and even though I called them friends, in truth, they weren't. Here is the test for it: do you feel worse after having hung out or spoken to certain people? You may have been having a great day, but something they said managed to bring you down, or you may have been having a bad day and they made you feel even worse.

    If there are people in your life that make you feel this way, I recommend minimising the amount of time you spend with them, or as I practise, cut them off completely. Sometimes, it's as simple as finding the people who make you feel happy and spending more time with them. Also, think about those who make you feel unhappy and spend as little time with them as possible.

2. **Train, exercise or meditate**
    This was a bit of a Catch 22 situation for me. For years, I used the gym and my training as an outlet, so they always acted as plasters that temporarily healed the problem. If I felt I was on the edge, I never dealt with it or asked myself who or what was making me

feel this way. I just went to the gym. I was effectively 'self-medicating' with exercise. In my opinion, it's actually the best way to reduce short, as well as long- term anxiety, but it's imperative to follow step one and then use training, exercise and meditation as ways to support you and not just put a lid over the real problem.

3. **Don't eat foods that make your anxiety worse**

This really could have been number one, but as it's discussed in more detail in the nutrition section, it is number three on the list.

I lacked self-awareness in my early twenties so much so that I never added two and two together in terms of how eating certain foods had a direct effect on my mood.

Knowing how certain foods can send my body into a spiral of 'fight or flight' has supported me massively over the past few years. If your body is intolerant or allergic to certain foods, or if you react to certain additives, flavourings and preservatives that can be found in heavily processed food, then it's worth keeping note of how you feel if these ingredients feature heavily in your diet.

For example, I know if I eat too much dairy, sugar or gluten, my brain will feel foggy the next day and I won't have the same steady energy and mood that I normally have. Everyone reacts differently to certain foods and ingredients, so experiment with it yourself.

I've largely eliminated these ingredients and foods and very rarely get any physiological anxiety issues anymore. If you still find yourself getting edgy and anxious for no apparent reason – it's not about money, a relationship or a job and you just feel 'off' – then I highly recommend having a look at your nutrition and checking if certain foods you consume are causing you to feel this way. See the nutrition section of the book for more on this.

CHAPTER 10
WORRY

How to crowd worry out of your mind

I think worry and anxiety are two sides of the same coin – we are the only species that have acquired the capacity to envision and anticipate our future. We also have what's called 'theory of mind', where I can think about what you're thinking about.

This can be an incredible thing – envisioning your future can allow you to create and be the architect of the lifestyle you wish to lead. Your theory of mind helps build incredible relationships with other people – the relationships that normally thrive are those where you can perceive the other person's point of view, or figuratively, 'put yourself in their shoes'.

Our brain, specifically our pre-frontal cortex, has

evolved to do this, but it also means that the same visionary mechanism can have opposite and negative effects if we don't manage it. Your brain is like a Rottweiler guard dog – if you mind it, care for it and look after it, it will serve you for life, but if you mistreat it or don't look after it, it can attack you, harm you and even kill you.

So what does that kind of negativity look like? It all comes under the same umbrella of worry. Instead of focusing on creating your dream body, life or job, you worry that you might not look good enough, that you will never meet the right person, have enough money or that people may not like you.

There's an incredible chapter in the book *Social* by Harvard professor Matthew Lieberman, whereby they put people into an FMRI machine (Functional Magnetic Resonance Imaging) – like an MRI, but for your brain – which shows the section that lights up when we are left with our own thoughts. When patients undergo this procedure after having just performed a simple task and are then left to their own devices, the part of the brain that is responsible for social relationships lights up. It happens every time that we are not focused on a particular task.

This means that every second we don't work, or when

we are engaged in a conversation or focusing on a task, our brain automatically starts thinking about our social relationships – the 'default mode'. Think about yourself. How often, as you've been driving home from work, have you replayed the conversations or interactions you had that day? 'What did Suzie mean by that comment?' or 'I wonder if Paul likes me?' We've all done it, and again, like most things, it constantly serves an evolutionary purpose. The more social awareness and theory of mind we possess, the more socially accepted we will be. Thousands of years ago, if you were isolated from your large hunter-gatherer group, it meant you ended up as dinner for some sabre-toothed tiger, so it was important to be accepted into the group.

This may explain why we have such a yearning to be liked and accepted. It's an evolutionary survival adaption. Like most things, when used positively, it can enhance your life tremendously. Deep down, most of us want to be accepted and liked by our peers and build positive and thriving relationships with people.

But what happens when the desire to socialize isn't positively channelled? Those social thoughts that allow us to integrate better into a society can consume every free moment, which leads to... you guessed it – worry!

So, the question is, how can I use this information to

support my own life? As someone who has spent a large portion of his life dealing with anxiety and worry, my story and learning tips from it will hopefully support you in moving forward.

Crying into a steering wheel until the penny finally drops

I will never forget the night when I nearly reached my breaking point. It was a few months before my daughter Holly was born and I had just finished working with twelve clients back-to-back. I was also preparing myself for the Fitness Model World Championships in Las Vegas. I had trained twice that day. I had more or less given up sleep at this stage, and my anxiety and worry were at an all-time high. Whenever I got the time to think, I would regularly ask myself, 'What if I didn't make the show? What if there is something wrong with my baby? What if I can't keep my business thriving? All fear and worry.

I love the acronym of FEAR: False Evidence Appearing Real. Here's why. I had worked myself up into a frenzy and I remember parking outside my new home and crying while simultaneously hitting my head on the steering wheel for what felt like an eternity.

My body felt encased in a vice while the jaws were

being drawn tighter and tighter. All my worries and fears felt very real at the time, but looking back, they were all illusions that I had created. My brain was over-thinking everything that could possibly go wrong. I've since created strategies, discussed below, that support me when any worries or fear feel like they are taking control of my body or mind.

Socrates says, 'know thyself', and one of the greatest gifts that I will be forever grateful for is my ability to see things before they actually happen in the context of my own life.

I trained myself in this ability when I played top-level sports, when I travelled the world as a professional fitness model and when I left the teaching profession to start my own business that served people better and on a much larger scale.

My own philosophy in life that has supported me greatly over the years is, 'Become the person you want to be and then wait for reality to catch up with that version of you'. I wanted to be a professional fitness model who travelled the world, so I acted, lived and became that person until reality caught up to me.

I wanted to create a business and a life that would help to serve as many people as possible, and I have tried my best to become that person. My biggest goal in life is to leave the world better than how I had found it, and to instil my life's philosophy into my daughter so that if she chooses to stand on the shoulders of giants, she has the character and a belief in herself to do it. I want the world to be better because we were here.

Sometimes, we determine our character by what we have or do, and that allows us to become that person. For example, if I have a nice car or a big house, then I will be successful, or if I do well in this show, test or exam, I can become successful.

In my opinion, the sequence of actions in that model is wrong. It's the 'do, have and be' model. If I do or have this, I can be that.

I think a better way to live life is by the 'be, do and have' model – if I can be this person, then I can do that and I'll have this. If you want to be in a better shape, you need to become a person who makes better food choices and creates better habits that support that end vision. Become a fit person in your mind, do things like eating well, creating supportive habits accordingly and exercising more. Be, do and have.

The ability to see into my future in the context of my own life has been one of my biggest drivers throughout my life. That night was an example: staring into my steering wheel, contemplating why I felt this was my turning point.

As I sat in the car feeling horribly sorry for myself, I looked into my audio book library and re-listened to one of my favourites: *Mastery* by Robert Greene. Suddenly, I felt as if a huge load was lifted from me. I was deeply engrossed in the book, and I felt free, if only for a short period of time. This was when I discovered my first trick to dealing with worry, which I call 'taking control of your free time', which ultimately is your thinking time.

Take control of your thinking time

The biggest difference in my life over the last two years, alongside the birth of my daughter, is my ability to take control of my wandering and unhelpful thoughts. Two years ago, if I were left to my own devices, my mind would wander off to the social interaction conversations I had that day, and my life never really changed. I had the same income, the same shape of mind and body, the same network of people I hung around with – nothing ever really progressed.

Now, I spend all my thinking time with audio books, podcasts or media that supports my end goal in all the areas of my life. I consume information that helps me on my own journey. I know that philosophy helps strengthen my mindset, so I read Seneca or Marcus Aurelius before bed. I know that reading books, going to seminars and doing courses on physiology, biomechanics and nutrition allow me to build my own knowledge that can directly impact the people I work with.

My advice would be to make a list of all the things you want in your life – the body you want, the job you want, the relationships you want – and put them all somewhere visible, where you can see them. After that, consume as much information as you can that supports that end goal. When I wanted to build my own body, I read every book and magazine that I could find that would support the image that I wanted to create. Sixteen years later, I have the body that I dreamed of having when I was thirteen years old.

Use your free time to consume the information that supports you in creating the life that you want. Before you know it, even when you are left to your own devices, your automatic thoughts start to manifest themselves in ways that support your vision– not to the silly comment made at you during lunchtime.

'What you think, you become.'

BUDDHA

When the worry is bigger

We have all had those near-breaking point moments, which look different for each person. It doesn't matter how big or small it appears to you – whether it's the death of a loved one or nasty words aimed in your direction by a colleague, it's all relative.

There are times when needless worry kicks in, and that's where taking control of your free-thinking time can serve you tremendously. However, if it's something that's continuously on your mind, you need to deal with it. I find that most of my worries tend to dissipate during my free-thinking time or when I exercise but there are times when it just keeps coming up again and again.

So many people relegate their thoughts to, 'It's not important', 'Nobody understands' or even worse, 'Nobody cares anyways', but the reality is that it's relative. No worry is too small – worries are like seeds – if that seed is planted and you leave it alone, it can grow into a mighty oak tree. Now ask yourself, what's easier – taking a bad seed from the ground or cutting down a massive oak tree? Next time you think, 'I'll just forget about it, it's nothing', think about that analogy.

Sometimes you just can't avoid the conflict

I think conflict avoidance is one the biggest detriments to happiness and has been the biggest factor in my own life for dealing with chronic worry. I know that time and again, I've figuratively built mountains out of mole hills by avoiding a conversation or a situation that I've built up in my own head. I avoided the conversation or the situation because I wanted to avoid the feeling of unease that I knew would inevitably come from it.

I would regularly avoid my inner conflict because of some story I had told myself to justify the situation: 'Oh I don't want to hurt this person's feelings' or 'It's probably not true anyway', etc. There were times when I just didn't want to admit that I was too much of a coward to take ownership of a situation.

Now, I like to think of tough words as workouts – all the growth and results come from leaning into the pain of the workout. If you are too comfortable when you work out, your body never really changes. You need to go outside of your comfort zone.

'The comfort zone is a beautiful place,
but nothing ever grows there.'

VINCENT VAN GOGH

In the gym, your body responds by losing more body fat or building more muscle. But when you deal with worry, your mind responds by making you much happier. If you are worried about something right now and it keeps coming up again and again, what conversation or situation are you avoiding? That's probably the one you need to have in order to rid yourself of chronic worry.

CHAPTER 11
PRACTICAL LIFE TIPS

I have, by no means, figured life out yet, and truthfully, I don't think anybody ever does, but that doesn't mean you can't strive to get everything you want. There are a few practical tips that have massively supported me in my life, so I'm going to share them with you.

Think with the end in mind

I remember listening to Stephen R Covey's 7 *Habits of Highly Effective People* audio book, from which one section has always stuck out in my mind.

He talks about seeing oneself going to the funeral of a loved one. Picture yourself driving to the funeral parlour or chapel, parking the car and getting out. As you walk inside the building, you notice the flowers and the organ music. You see the faces of friends and family passing along the way. As you walk down to the front of the room and look inside the coffin, you suddenly come face to face with yourself. This is *your* funeral, three years from today. All these people have come to honour you, to express feelings of love and appreciation for your life. As you wait for the service to begin, you see that there are four speakers. The first is from your family – children, parents, aunts, uncles, nieces' nephews. The second is one of your friends, someone who knew you closely as a person. The third is from your work or profession, and the fourth is someone you were involved with from your community. Now think deeply. What would you like each of these speakers to say about you and your life?

This section struck me more than anything else in the entire book. I remember walking towards my apartment in East London. The streetlights were lit and it was a cold, frosty November night. I stopped dead in my tracks to contemplate what I had just listened to.

The vision that painted in my mind was so clear and vivid that it hit me like a ton of bricks. It also dawned on me that I wasn't happy with the answer to the question that was forming in my head. That was the moment I decided to leave London to pursue my passion. Shortly after, I left my job, moved back home with my parents (broke and on welfare) and tried to set up a new life, where my funeral would matter, where my life would matter. That was the day when my mind shifted from being content with life to the seed that was recently planted: 'I'm only going to get one life!'

> 'You only live once, but if you do
> it right, once is enough'
>
> **MAE WEST**

The most fundamental application of 'begin with the end in mind' is to begin today with the image or picture of your life and what you want it to look like. The funeral scenario is the most extreme of cases, but the paradigm or mind shift that I experienced that day stuck with me, and is now channelled into all aspects of my life.

By keeping that end clearly in mind, you can ensure that whatever you do on any particular day does not violate the criteria you have defined as supremely important, and that each day of your life contributes in a meaningful way to the vision you have of your life or as a whole. I once had a talk with a client of mine who was looking to excel as one of the top sporting athletes in the country and is currently on the brink of breaking into one of the top teams where fame and recognition would be guaranteed. We talked about beginning with the end in mind and working back from that. I always try to follow the 10% law: your goals and targets should be so high that even if you only hit 10% of it, you would have still achieved more than 99.9% of what you ever dreamed possible.

I mentioned this to my client. I told him that if he wanted to make it to that team, he would have to train, eat and live like the #1 athlete on the planet.

For example, when I competed at the 2015 World Fitness Model Championships in Las Vegas, I aimed to win the entire show and become #1 fitness model in the world. I trained, lived and made every decision as if I was already that person. I managed to finish eighth, which made me one of the top 10 competitors in the entire world. Had I aimed for top 10, I probably wouldn't have made the sacrifices necessary to move into that bracket.

> 'Aim for the moon,
> and you will at least
> hit the stars'
>
> **W. CLEMENT STONE**

Funnily enough, my daughter was born a couple of months before that show and my life took an entirely different direction: my health now became a priority – it wasn't just about me anymore. I now had a little girl who I always needed to be there for, and my lifestyle at the time didn't support that new vision. My daughter saved me from things that probably would have eventually affected my health. I started to think with a new end in mind.

Is what you're doing supporting the end goal?

I have three massive whiteboards in my bedroom. One has all my goals for the next 12 months, the other 24 months and the third, the next 10 years.

If I am ever worried or unsure about a decision I have to make, I look at those three boards and ask myself, 'Does this support the end goal?' If the answer is 'no', I don't do it; if the answer is 'yes', I go all out with it.

It's incredibly easy to get caught up in leading a busy life, to work harder and harder while climbing the ladder of success, only to discover that it's leaning against the wrong wall. The three whiteboards are my way of making sure that the decisions I make are effective in moving me up the ladder that's up against the right wall.

People often find themselves achieving victories that are empty – success that has come at the expense of things they suddenly realise were far more valuable to them. For example, one of my main goals in life that probably trumps all others is having a strong enough relationship with my daughter so that I become her 'go-to' person in life. My mum has always been my 'go-to' person and I want to be that person for my daughter. I know how to do this – I always need to be present with her.

Up until the last couple of years, too often, I would find myself taking out my phone, scrolling through social media while in the company of other people. What's worse is they would be doing the same and neither of us would see anything wrong in it.

I remember reading *The Will Power Instinct* by Kelly McGonigal, where she talks about how it takes willpower to say 'no' to things and how to be present with the people you care about the most. If you want a better relationship with someone, be it your partner, your parents or your children, be present when you are with them.

The book talks about a study done on husbands and fathers who were physically present at home for at least six hours a day, but spent the entire time either watching TV or working. In relative terms, this father or husband would be with his family for at least six hours, but he wasn't present for the majority or any of the six hours.

In contrast, the study looked at husbands and fathers who were only home for one hour a day but spent that entire hour engaging with their families. There was no TV turned on in the background and no scrolling through social media, just quality family time where there were no distractions or 'noise'.

Obviously, the familial relationships of the one-hour dads were much stronger than that of the six-hour dads, yet in relative terms, they spent much less time at home.

The difference? Being fully present.

My end goal is to always be there for my daughter and have a relationship with her, through which I can help steer her on her life's path. To build that kind of a relationship, I need to be present when I'm with her. This book is my own reminder and a device of accountability that should help me retain that vision.

How different our lives are when we really know what is deeply important to us, and keeping that picture in mind, we manage ourselves each day to be and do what really matters the most. Always keep the end goal in mind and work backwards from it. If the ladder is not leaning against the right wall, every step we take just gets us to the wrong place faster.

This can be applied to anything – I use the same techniques in my business, my fitness goals and my personal life. You wouldn't build a house without first creating every detail and blueprint before you hammer the first nail in place. Your life is the same. Create a blueprint for your life and then build the life you want.

Don't let negative people stop you

Something funny happens when you start moving in the direction of what truly drives you to build the life, body or relationships that you really want. Negativity from others starts to seep through.

This is something I've seen first-hand and personally struggled with. I even had the quote, 'The only taste of success some people get is when they take a bite out of you' posted on my wall for my first two years in business. This was my way of dealing with negative comments that used to rock me to my core.

You only have to go on social media to see some of

the hate aimed at successful people. Nobody kicks a dead dog, so if people are talking about you, hating or nay-saying – assuming you are not hurting, harming or neglecting people – it's probably a sign that you are moving in the right direction.

When I talk about negativity, I'm talking about comments and words coming from outside your immediate circle of friends. When I think about my circle, four names spring to mind immediately – people who have my back and I theirs, regardless of circumstances. Think about the three or four people, friends, family members or partners who have your back and then do everything in your power to continuously build and nurture those relationships. Provided they support you on becoming the best version of you, then their opinions matter – nobody else's does.

How to deal with people telling you that you can't do something

> 'There is nothing either good or bad, but thinking makes it so.'
>
> **WILLIAM SHAKESPEARE**

We choose how we look at things. We retain the ability to inject perspective into any given situation.

We can't change the obstacles or perceived bad things themselves – that part of the equation is set, but the power of perspectives can change how the obstacle or bad things appear.

As someone who puts his thoughts, opinions and life applications out there for the world to see, I leave myself open to criticism about my appearance, ideas or philosophies. A lot of these can be perceived as negative comments aimed in my direction.

> 'Say nothing,
> do nothing,
> be nothing.'
>
> **ARISTOTLE**

I made a choice a long time ago about how I would approach, view, and contextualize any of that criticism aimed at me – I decided it was up to me whether to accept it or not.

In every aspect of your life, it's your choice whether you want to put 'I' in front of something (I am angry with those comments, I am annoyed someone would say that, I am disappointed that person used those words). These add an extra element, which is 'you' in relation to the criticism, rather than the criticism itself. The criticism is not you and you are not the criticism. Those two things are separate, so let them go and don't let it consume your entire being. We go through our entire life worrying about what other people think and make decisions based out of fear because of what our parents, our friends or even strangers think!

When you try to please everyone, you end up pleasing no one.

With the wrong perspective, we get consumed and overwhelmed with something actually quite small. Through the readings of Seneca and other stoic philosophers, I can now see from the perspective that sometimes, the criticism or negativity aimed in our direction is actually the other person's way of consciously or subconsciously dealing with their own demons.

Remember that choosing to accept negativity is your decision

It took me a long time to realize that a lot of the negativity I aimed towards other people was a reflection of my inner self, which said more about me than the person I was aiming those emotions towards.

I remember a close friend doing me a bad turn once. I hold

loyalty and respect as two of the main characteristics in my closest network and 'talking behind someone's back' or to put it simply, 'being two-faced', is probably the least desirable characteristic a person can have in my opinion. Listening to destructive comments and negative stories from people who were supposed to be your closest friends can be a difficult reality to process – it can lead to a lot of built-up hate and trust issues.

Luckily, those circumstances can make you considerably stronger and more self-aware if you allow a shift in perspective. Off the back end of that particular situation, two things happened:

It allowed me to really figure what kind of people I wanted in my life and what I valued most in others. I now have an inner circle of people who I trust with my life. Jack Canfield says in his book *The 20 Success Principles* that 'success leaves clues', but I think failures leave just as many – you probably learn even more from your failures and bad experiences.

I also realized that those negative feelings or 'hate' were emotions that had to originate within me for it to be even aimed in the direction of another person. That particular situation allowed me to search for my own inner hate and made me ask the question, 'What was it that I hated about myself that was manifesting itself in my feelings toward another person?'

The motivational speaker Tony Robbins regularly talks about the power of questions. In this circumstance, I asked the right questions and I found the right answers. I realized that it was my own demons that I had to first deal with before I could release the hate or negative feelings towards another person. Now when I feel moments of hate towards someone, something or some idea, I recognize it for what it is – just an emotion. So I let it in, allowing myself to feel it and then let it go.

> 'Hating someone
> is like drinking poison
> and then expecting the
> other person to die.'
>
> **BUDDHA**

Words are thoughts and ideas, not bullets

As mentioned above, hate is something that has to be within you in order for you to project it onto somebody else; how to deal with it is down to how you see it. My closest friends have referred to me on several occasions as 'bulletproof' when they see negative comments and words aimed in my direction. I'm not bulletproof – the reality is, I see words as thoughts and ideas and not bullets.

For one, thoughts and ideas change – my philosophies, opinions and entire perspective on life is considerably different now than it was five or ten years ago. Any negativity aimed in your direction goes with the moment. Every moment is a new moment.

Sometimes, people hold onto the ideas and thoughts that may have held weight in that particular moment in time, but that moment is temporary.

I remember family members telling me how stupid I was for leaving my teaching job and trying to start my own business. Years later, the very same people now talk about how they knew I was going to make it – the circumstances changed, more information was now available. Enough time had passed so that their subjective vision of success was now perceived to have been achieved, and their opinions had changed.

The original 'You're stupid' was now forgotten, relegated to non-existence in the past and replaced with 'I knew you could do it'. This is how people are. Those thoughts and opinions are held for a moment in time and people can change them with the turning of the tide – normally, when more evidence is given to support or negate the idea but it is still just an opinion, an idea.

We as an entire species once knew the world was flat but Aristotle argued that the earth was spherical, because of the circular shadow it cast on the moon during a lunar eclipse. We now know that the earth is round.

'Everything we hear
is an opinion, not a fact.
Everything we see is perspective,
not the truth'

MARCUS AURELIUS

But when these thoughts and opinions are aimed in our direction, we consciously or subconsciously hold on to it like our first-born child! Realizing that every word that's ever been aimed in your direction is an opinion of that moment in time can liberate you to do anything in your life. The thoughts you have in your own head are what count. If you let other people's words dictate the direction of your life, you will never get what you want.

When you start to see the world and all the opinions and thoughts in it as simply a perspective, it can liberate you like nothing else.

Opinions and thoughts are what are felt in that moment, they're not bullets – they're words thrown into the air

– not even words cemented in stone. They're mostly words that float in air that we take in and allow to dictate the direction of our lives.

It's nice to hear people refer to you as 'bulletproof', but again this is just an opinion of that particular moment – when you give words less weight, the damage they do becomes a moot point.

One of the reasons I love my life is that regardless of the negative or positive comments aimed in my direction, I'm going to continue to do what I'm doing and just, 'do me'. When you can truly let go of the thoughts and opinions because that's all they are, the world will be your oyster. Just 'do you' and be happy.

CHAPTER 12
TEN LIFE LESSONS

'Smart people learn from their mistakes. But the real sharp ones learn from the mistakes of others.'

BRANDON MULL

I remember the penny dropping when I heard this quote for the first time. I was listening to one of my mentors and how they read books to learn from other people's mistakes.

I remember thinking, 'I can literally delve into the mind of some of the world's greatest thinkers and actually see their thoughts'. For a long time, I believed that thoughts become things. This was the moment when I went to seek out some of the world's greatest thinkers to try and influence the inner workings of my own mind.

As a child with a love of sport, I would spend hours copying and replicating the moves of my favourite footballers and soccer players – this would be no different.

Instead of trying to solo off one foot and shoot with the other like the football star Pat Spillane or step over and back-heel a pass like the soccer prodigy Zinedine Zidane, I would practice using the mental strategies and techniques that have supported some of the greatest thinkers in history to strengthen and improve my own mind and my own conscience (and subconscious) thoughts.

That's when I learnt about Confucius.

> 'When the student is ready,
> the teacher will appear.'
>
> **BUDDHA**

Confucius was, in my opinion, the greatest Eastern philosopher of all time, whose teachings deeply influenced East Asian life and thought.

He is considered China's first teacher and his teachings are usually expressed in short phrases which are open to various interpretations. Chief among his philosophical ideas is the importance of a virtuous life, filial piety (respecting parents and elders) and ancestral study.

In Yu Dan's book *Confucius From The Heart*, he talks about the necessity for benevolent, kind and frugal rulers, the importance of inner moral harmony and its direct connection with harmony in the physical world and how rulers and teachers are important role models for the wider society.

Sometimes when reading, I make notes of the things that come up that will either lead to a blog post, a podcast or some other medium where I think others may benefit from what I've read. This is what came up for me and I've included it as the last section of this book as it's something I still read every single morning. I hope it helps.

ONE WHEREVER YOU DECIDE TO GO, GO 100%

I have no regrets in life. I honestly believe that all the bad stuff and things you would take back if you could, have merged the character of who you are today.

That being said, one of the life advices I would give my younger self would be, 'Once you know what you want, go after it with all of your heart'. I make all my life decisions on the simple premise that it's either a 'Hell, yes' or it's a 'No'. If it doesn't excite me, I don't do it. If it does, I'm all in.

TWO EVERYTHING AND EVERYONE HAS BEAUTY, BUT NOT EVERYONE SEES IT

I have been a victim of this in the past. If someone has annoyed me or been rude to me (rudeness is one of my biggest pet peeves), I have labelled them as 'being rude'. Rudeness, like most things that annoy us, is an action, not a characteristic. Only when

I learnt to separate the thoughts of what they're doing as an action and not who they are, was I able to detach myself and realize that some people are just having a bad day and it's not a reflection on their character – and definitely not a reflection on you.

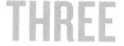 IT DOES NOT MATTER HOW SLOWLY YOU GO, AS LONG AS YOU DON'T STOP

> 'Only dead fish go with the flow.'
>
> **ANDY HUNT**

It doesn't matter how slowly you are moving forward toward the life, mind or body you want, as long as you're moving in the right direction and 'have the ladder up against the right wall', you will eventually get to where you want to be. Remember Aesop's

fable of the tortoise and the hare – slow and steady wins the race.

FOUR IF YOU THINK YOU HAVE ALL THE ANSWERS, YOU HAVEN'T ASKED ALL THE QUESTIONS

One of the miraculous beauties of life is that we will never know it all. Things change, ideas change, science changes – we are creatures constantly evolving.

Around 330 BC, Aristotle maintained on the basis of physical theory and observational evidence that the Earth was spherical (round) and reported on an estimate on the circumference. Up until that point, we knew the world was flat – just think about that whenever you think you know something.

FIVE LIFE IS REALLY SIMPLE, BUT WE INSIST ON MAKING IT COMPLICATED

Find the things that make you happy, do more of it. Find the things that make you unhappy, do less of it.

SIX IF YOU HATE SOMEBODY, THAT'S ON YOU, NOT THEM

Hate is a horrible thing to be consumed by, and it's a basic human feeling.

Hate, like every other human emotion, is nothing more than a manifestation of thought – you control it. Hate puts your mind into a negative place, where the mere association of the person you associate this feeling with can destroy you as a person and your underlying happiness.

Are there people I dislike? Of course! But hate, that's an emotion I try and keep out of my conscience and subconscious. 'If it doesn't support you, get rid of it" – that feeling supports very few people and those that it did (Hitler, Stalin and Mussolini to name a few), well, you know what happened there.

SEVEN DON'T ADJUST THE GOALS, ADJUST THE ACTION STEPS

'If your dreams don't scare you,
they aren't big enough.'

ELLEN JOHNSON SIRLEAF

As human beings, we have put a man on the moon. We physically designed a piece of machinery that could leave our atmosphere and go to another planet.

Sam Walton (the creator of Walmart Stores) was worth 160 billion dollars when he died – that's one hundred and sixty thousand million dollars. Are you telling me Sam Walton is one hundred and sixty thousand million times smarter than you? I didn't think so.

Next time you try to 'get down four dress sizes' or 'get abs for the summer' and wonder if you can do it, remember that as a species, we have put a man on the moon. Aim small, miss small.

EIGHT RESPECT YOURSELF AND OTHERS WILL RESPECT YOU

One of my biggest goals in life is to instil the feeling of self-worth and respect into my daughter. I would trade every single thing in my life to make sure my girl grows up with confidence and self-respect.

I truly believe that respecting yourself gives you the confidence to be truly happy in life. How can anybody else respect you if you don't respect yourself?

NINE WHAT THE HAPPY PERSON LOOKS FOR IN THEMSELVES, THE UNHAPPY PERSON LOOKS FOR IN OTHERS

Happiness comes from within, it's not a tangible thing. A nice car, a new house, an attractive partner – none of these things in themselves bring true 'happiness' or 'fulfilment'. They're external sources that can be taken away with a blink of an eye.

Sure, they're nice for a little while and your ego will happily take the nice comments, but again, those sweet comments are simply words from other people. If other people's comments are what's making you happy, then you're always going to need something external or superficial to retain that happiness.

Learn to find the happiness from within and you will always be happy.

 # STUDY THE PAST IF YOU WANT TO DEFINE THE FUTURE

'There is no such thing as a new problem,
the answer is written down
– you just need to find it.'

In conclusion, learning from other people's mistakes or triumphs can allow you to create any life that you want. As someone who has struggled with energy, sleep, getting in shape and anxiety, amongst other things, and came out the other side stronger because of it, I hope this books serves as a blueprint to cut your own learning curve.

Remember that thoughts become things – the ideas you put into your head become the thoughts that you have, and your thoughts influence actions. The actions you take dictate the direction of your life. Decide who you want to be and build your life around becoming that person.

If you want to have more energy, sleep better, have the body you always wanted, or be the person who has the confidence to stand tall in any room, then consume every bit of information that supports that vision. I hope this book has helped to support you on that journey. Please share it with your friends or family who you feel will benefit from it as well.

I'll leave you all with one final quote that I think sums up this entire section of the book.

> 'When writing the story of your own life, don't let somebody else hold the pen.'
>
> **HARLEY DAVIDSON**

ACKNOWLEDGEMENTS

My gratitude goes out to all those who have passed through my life. All of you have contributed in some way to my journey and the substance of this book.

First, I want to thank my publisher Lucy McCarraher and Rethink Press. Without them, this book would not be possible.

My father Gerry, who has supported me through my entire life and nurtured a work ethic that still supports me to this day.

My sister Karen, who has always been my second biggest fan in everything that I do. She has been one of my best friends and is one of the smartest people I've had the pleasure of knowing.

My team of Paul Dermody, Daniel Lupton and Emma Finnegan – while writing this book, Paul,

Daniel and Emma allowed me to bounce ideas off them on a daily basis and really helped the book take a certain direction. I couldn't have completed this book without their support.

Finally, to whom this book is dedicated – my mum Rita and my daughter Holly. My mum and my daughter are the two closest people in my life. The reason I couldn't pick one or the other is because without either, there would be no book. Without my mum, I wouldn't be on my current journey and have the mindset that I have, and without Holly, I wouldn't have my 'why'.

This book is dedicated to them, for without them, I would not be the man, son or father I am today. I love you both.

Thank you.

RECOMMENDED RESOURCES

Bonus video downloads

The training program videos are on www.briankeanefitness.com. You can download the videos that go through the entire workout and on how to perform each move correctly.

THE AUTHOR

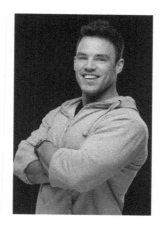

BRIAN KEANE

Brian is an online fitness trainer; former professional fitness model and the owner of Brian Keane Fitness. He and his team help serve thousands of people each year through their online fitness programs.

Brian's fitness journey started when his parents bought him a gym membership for his 16th birthday. He has been training ever since.

He also worked as a primary school teacher for four years whilst setting up a personal training business on the side. In 2014, he left the teaching profession to pursue a full-time career in fitness and in the same year he won his Fitness Model Pro Card at the Miami Pro Event. He spent nearly two years traveling the world as an international fitness model before his daughter was born on 25th of May 2015.

Since then, Brian has dedicated all of his time to his daughter and building a business that serves people on a global scale.

His BKF Online Fat Loss and Muscle Building Program specialises in getting people into shape through finding nutritional strategies that work for each person and using short high intensity training sessions that fits it into each person's lifestyle and schedule.

The graduates of the program range from stay at home moms, athletes and everyday gym goers, to first time trainers, factory workers and business executives.

Brian's #1 rated podcast is now one of the most recognized health and fitness podcasts in the Irish and UK market and his social media presences in growing into the hundreds of thousands across all platforms at the time of print. To find out more about Brian, check out the links below.

Website: www.briankeanefitness.com
Facebook: Brian Keane Fitness
YouTube: Brian Keane Fitness
Instagram: brian_keane_fitness
Snapchat: briank019
Podcast: The Brian Keane Fitness Podcast

Lightning Source UK Ltd.
Milton Keynes UK
UKHW02f2156050418
320594UK00016B/388/P